STREET CRAZY

The Tragedy of the Homeless Mentally Ill

Stephen B. Seager M.D.

WESTCOM PRESS

Publisher: WESTCOM PRESS
2110 Artesia Boulevard, Suite 183
Redondo Beach, CA 90278
Phone: (310) 374-0988
Fax: (310) 371-8244
Web: http://www.StreetCrazy.com

Publisher's Cataloging-in-Publication
Seager, Stephen B.
Street Crazy : the tragedy of the homeless mentally ill / Stephen B. Seager M.D.
p. cm.
ISBN: 0-9665827-7-2
Current Affairs.

Library of Congress Catalog Card Number: 98-86873

Book Design & Typesetting: SageBrush Publications, Tempe, Arizona
Printing: McNaughton & Gunn, Inc. Saline, Michigan

Dedication

To Shannan, Jim, Brett and Stevie.

To Michael and Nancy.

Most of all, to sweet Mia Kay.

You are loved.

Acknowledgements

I wish to respectfully thank the following people for their gracious and generous assistance in the preparation of this book.

The Honorable Barry Perrou Psy.D. Commissioner, Department of Mental Health, Los Angeles County. Commander, Los Angeles County Sheriff's Department.

The Honorable Harold Shabo, Supervising Judge, Mental Health Department, Los Angeles County Superior Court.

The Honorable Richard Vagnozzi, Deputy District Attorney, Los Angeles County District Attorney's Office, Psychiatric Division.

The Honorable Melvin Higashi, Deputy Public Defender, Los Angeles County Public Defenders Office.

The Honorable Laurie Gelfand, Deputy District Attorney, Los Angeles County District Attorney's Office, Psychiatric Division.

Sandra Krause, Court Manager, Office of Counselor in Mental Health, Los Angeles County Superior Court.

Michael Frane, Office of Counselor in Mental Health, Hearing Officer.

Patricia Gilbert Ph.D., Patients' Rights Advocate Office, Los Angeles County Department of Mental Health.

Carla Jacobs, California Alliance for the Mentally Ill

Milton Miller M.D., Chairman, Department of Psychiatry, Harbor/UCLA Medical Center. Professor, Department of Psychiatry, UCLA School of Medicine. Acting Medical Director, Department of Mental Health, Los Angeles County. You are a mentor and friend.

J. Richard Elpers M.D., Professor of Psychiatry, UCLA School of Medicine. Outpatient Director, Harbor/UCLA Medical Center. Past Medical Director, Department of Mental Health, Los Angeles County. You sparked a young psychiatrist's interest in the history of his profession.

Florence Feiler, an agent who has gone beyond the bounds of professional assistance. You are family.

Mette Hansen M.D., UCLA Medical Center. For incisive, unwavering and voluminous editorial assistance. For a personal commitment of time far beyond anything anyone has a right to expect. For agonizing over and enjoying the experience with me. For, literally, teaching me, step by step, to become a better writer. It's your book as much as mine. There aren't thanks enough.

Richard Sabaroff, for typing assistance.

Contents

 # Introduction

"WHERE DO YOU LIVE, MR. SMITH?" asked the public defender, a slight woman with a determined face.

Mr. Smith shifted a bit in the witness chair. His thinning hair was long and bedraggled. Three deep, partially healed wounds ran down his right cheek. "Underneath a car," he said.

"Where is that car located?"

"Vacant lot."

"Do you know the address of the lot?"

"Santa Monica."

"This vehicle provides you with adequate protection from the rain?"

"It's a good car." Mr. Smith leaned back. "Been there for..."

"And what do you eat?" the attorney persisted.

"I know rancid garbage. Don't touch that," Mr. Smith replied. "Maggots are from God. They tell me what's bad."

The attorney, seated behind a long table before an imposing judicial bench, looked up. "Then you know which food in the garbage is good and which is bad?"

"Yes, the maggots..."

"Do you plan to kill yourself or anyone else?" the attorney interrupted.

Mr. Smith paused, cocking his head. "Been shot twice already. Don't think God or the maggots want that."

"Thank you, Mr. Smith," the attorney said, apparently satisfied. "Your witness."

I sat in the audience section of the courtroom, second row next to the center aisle. I'd already testified. It was my third day as a psychiatrist-in-training. Mr. Smith was the first patient I'd taken to court to detain for further treatment. He'd come to our facility five days earlier having been found at the bottom of a drainage ditch soaking wet, babbling and bleeding. According to passers-by, a pack of feral dogs had mauled him. Not spotted, he would have died during the night.

Despite our ministrations, Mr. Smith still looked terrible. Save one molar and incisor on the left, his mouth was toothless. Our clean hospital clothing hung on a skeletal frame like dropcloths over attic furniture. A leg infection was barely beginning to heal. The facial lacerations, recently scabbed over, would cause permanent scarring. Mr. Smith was fifty-six years old, had been homeless for fifteen years and suffered from chronic schizophrenia.

The district attorney, representing the hospital, stood. "Do you think living under a car is appropriate shelter?" he asked.

"Shit, yes," Mr. Smith said.

"And eating garbage gives you enough nutrition?"

"I've been sick some but ain't died so far. No maggots in me." He grinned crookedly.

"No further questions," the D.A. said.

The courtroom fell silent as the judge pondered his decision.

"It's dry underneath the car?" he finally asked Mr. Smith.

"No maggots, no rain. Dry as a bone," Mr. Smith answered.

"And food with maggots is bad. You know that?" the judge continued.

"All maggots are bad," Mr. Smith replied confidently.

"Thank you, Mr. Smith."

After another pause, the judge began speaking again. "Mr. Smith has demonstrated that he can provide himself with shelter and food. He's not dangerous. The writ is granted. The hospital's hold is released. You're free to go, Mr. Smith."

Mr. Smith rose, mumbled something over his shoulder, hobbled past the spectators and out the door. Back to the streets.

My jaw dropped. I had thought the decision to keep Mr. Smith hospitalized had been so obvious. Watching that ragged man limp away, I could no longer contain myself. "He'll die out there," I blurted at the psychiatrist sitting beside me, a middle-aged woman preparing to testify in the next mental health hearing. She didn't look over.

"Probably so," she said.

"I don't get this."

"No one does," she replied.

II

In some form, this scene is re-enacted daily in American courtrooms. Across the nation, scores of mentally sick persons are judicially removed from hospitals and let out into the streets to care for themselves despite repeated episodes demonstrating that they clearly can't do this.

We all know these people—the homeless mentally ill. They've become a fixture of our national urban landscape. We see them in parks and subway tunnels, sleeping on steam grates or sprawled across the sidewalk. These are the individuals loudly rambling to no one in particular, rank with their own excrement, wandering in traffic.

Not all homeless people are mentally ill. Some are drug addicts, others choose to live as they do. Many are on the street due to economic circumstance. These aren't the people about whom I'm talking. I'm concerned with the ones who are homeless because they're sick. According to different sources, one-third to one-half of the homeless population is chronically mentally ill. That's roughly one million people.

We're moved by them. We feel guilt over their predicament. We fear them. But few of us know why they behave and live as they do. And most are confused when it comes to assisting them in any significant way.

I hope to change this situation. By explaining our current understanding concerning the cause of mental illness, by demonstrating how the present treatment system functions and why it developed, this book aims to illuminate a bit of the darkness surrounding mental illness in America. A human story at heart, it's a look at the murky, dangerous world of the seriously mentally ill told by someone from the inside.

I intend to illustrate how grave mental illness affects not only the people who suffer from its devastation but also the impact it has on their families and those who try to treat these diseases. Mental illness touches nearly every American family. Yet, this is a subject about which very few people talk. We don't understand and thus are alarmed by it, oftentimes thinking that, if ignored, perhaps it, and those disturbing people, will go away.

Fear has always been a natural reaction to serious mental disease, but it needn't be so. We simply need the answer to certain questions. Who are these people? What afflicts them? Might I catch it? Can they be helped? These are quandaries that have generated discussion for thousands of years. We're certainly not the first ones to be troubled by them.

Mental illness isn't new to the twentieth century nor is our dread of it. These maladies have always been with us, as ancient as history itself. In order to alleviate our terror, we have developed various conflicting hypotheses to explain mental disease. The controversy has classically revolved around its cause. Three ideas have permeated this debate. (1) Are mental afflictions supernatural in origin, either a divine punishment for sin, or the doings of nefarious beings, namely demons and witches? (2) Could their genesis be a bad environment, improper parenting, life stress or the eruption of a Freudian Id into consciousness—the so-called "psychological" theories? Or (3) are they (as was first posited by the ancient Greeks) simply disorders of the brain, no more mystical than any other biological ailment? From century to century, each view has had its proponents.

The debate, however, is now over. With the advent of modern brain scanning machines and other sophisticated scientific techniques, the mental illnesses have proven to be diseases of the brain. Nothing more, nothing less. Mental illness is a problem with the brain, as heart disease is a problem with the heart. They aren't other-worldly or psychological.

What, then, are these brain afflictions? Why do they force people to live in the streets? There are many so-called mental disorders, but, based on severity of symptoms and the amount of havoc they wreck in a person's life, three stand out from the rest: major depression, bipolar disorder and schizophrenia. When discussing the homeless mentally ill, they're almost always diagnosed with one of these three syndromes in ascending order of frequency.

Major depression consists of long bouts of profoundly sad mood combined with feelings of hopelessness, chronic fatigue, changes in weight, poor concentration, irritability, interrupted sleep and, unfortunately, thoughts of self-destruction. The preponderance of people who commit suicide suffer from untreated depression.

While the exact cause of depression remains unclear, evidence points toward a decline in the function of serotonin. This is one of a class of chemicals called "neurotransmitters," molecules brain cells use to communicate with each other. The newer anti-depressants—Prozac, Paxil, Zoloft and the like—selectively increase the function of cerebral serotonin and relieve the symptoms of this disease.

Most people with depression get completely well or nearly so with adequate anti-depressant treatment, but a few do not. For them, the medications are intolerable or simply don't work. The resulting long bouts of melancholy eventually alienate these individuals from family and friends, the person's job becomes difficult to handle, and chronic debility results. A group of people with unrelenting depression ends up on the streets but in relatively small numbers.

Manic depression, or what's now coined as "bipolar disorder," is akin to major depression. The two are called "Mood Disorders." Those who suffer from bipolar disorder have the same prolonged bouts of depression but also periods of mania, the opposite of depression. Bursting with energy, some don't sleep for days on end. Rather than feeling hopeless, they assume they are capable of performing incredible, super-human feats or have been transformed into business tycoons, the President and, traditionally, Napoleon.

Instead of blackness, a manic person sees bright splurging colors. Imagining himself to be wealthy beyond belief and acting accordingly, a manic person may find a bill for three-hundred thousand dollars on his American Express card statement.

Mania is a frequent cause of psychosis—hearing voices, believing things that are patently not true or using grossly disordered thinking—which leads these unfortunate folks to perform outlandish, violent and sometimes disastrous acts.

Not always euphoric, "bipolars," as they're called, can tip over into extreme irritability as well, often becoming belligerent, fighting with the police or family members. Infused with omnipotent powers, they rarely brook criticism or restraint.

The devastation wrought by bipolars can be unbelievable. In the throes of a manic run, some will have sex with multiple anonymous partners thus ruining long, stable marriages. They will get AIDS. A carefully tended family business will be ruined. Bar brawls can eventuate in prison time.

Interestingly, a current explanation for bipolar disorder is that it may be a variety of epilepsy. The most effective treatments for mania are anti-seizure medications, e.g., Depakote, Tegretol, Neurontin and Lamictal. The old standby, lithium, is gradually passing out of favor, mainly due to unpleasant side effects.

On the correct dose of medicine, the greater number of people with bipolar disorder can also live normal or nearly normal lives.

Sometimes, however, these people don't feel the need for help. And, again, for a percentage, side effects of the remedy are unpleasant. This leads to unmanaged disease and possible marital, financial or employment disaster. Five to ten percent of the homeless mentally ill suffer from brittle bipolar disease.

Schizophrenia is, unfortunately, another story. People who contract this disastrous condition make up a vast majority of the homeless mentally ill, consigned by sickness to an agonizing life and early death. They're the people this book is mainly about.

Why do people with schizophrenia live on the street? The answer has roots as far back as the Greek philosophers Plato and Aristotle. It runs through Ancient Rome, the Middle Ages, the Renaissance,

Nineteenth Century Idealism and the 1960s' radical social revolution. The tale is strange and circuitous. It involves religion, human nature, medicine and the law.

Sadly, very few people know this story. We just see the results. In our hearts, we recognize something is wrong but aren't quite sure what. We're not, as I've discovered, alone in this feeling. Despite the staggering medical and human cost, most doctors can't fathom how the mentally ill came to be homeless. It's not taught in medical schools. Remarkably, even the bulk of psychiatrists, medical specialists that treat these diseases, don't comprehend why either.

Few judges and lawyers who deal daily with the homeless mentally ill are conversant with the facts, nor are many politicians and other decisions makers. Why, then, would the average citizen understand? We have a dilemma acknowledged by everyone but about which people know very little.

This book will attempt to change that. The antidote for fear is knowledge. I hope to present the seriously mentally ill as real people who have become ill, people deserving of our understanding and compassion, not aversion and neglect. I would like to have you ponder, contemplate and then, perhaps, take action. As we shall see, despite the apparent enormity of the problem, we actually have resolved this dilemma before and can again if we only care to consider it.

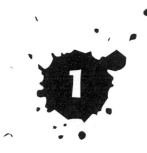

1 Of Lice and Men

"HE'S A STREET DING. Calls himself John Doe. Been here a thousand times," explained Tom "Bull" Willis, former Marine drill sergeant, now head nurse, walking alongside two policemen as they escorted a tattered piece of human refuse in through the front doors of our Los Angeles County psychiatric emergency department. The cops, bracketing the shuffling wretch and nudging him forward, could barely contain their disgust. One finally broke away, burying his nose in a sleeve. I thought he was going to vomit. It wouldn't have been the first time.

"Found him wandering down the 91 freeway," the other cop said, turning his head to the side as well.

"Let's hose him!" Bull boomed, waving toward me and Bill Ten-Trees, a stocky Navajo nursing attendant.

"Not again," I sighed after recognizing our new charge. We hustled over and took John Doe from the relieved cops then quickly walked toward the back door.

Though the man had been in the ER only briefly, his smell seeped everywhere.

"Jesus Christ?!" Dr. Andrew Yang, an intern, popped his head out of the doctors lounge.

"Did someone shit?" Dr. Alice Dupree, a second year resident-in-training, shouted from inside an exam cubicle. Her question wasn't meant to be discourteous. Where we worked, shit was a daily fact of life.

Even the patients in our holding room, a score of muttering people lost in their own tortured world of psychosis, began to bang on the observation window.

The odor was more than that of excrement. It was the smell of the sewer. Of disease. Of rot. Unless you've experienced it, you just can't know. Distinctly indescribable, it must be, I've concluded, something akin to the stench that leads detectives to long dead bodies stuffed into the trunks of abandoned cars.

Once outside, I grabbed a garden hose from the pavement. With me at the spigot and Bull at the nozzle, we hosed down John Doe until enough dirt, filth and vermin had been removed to reveal some semblance of a human form.

"He gets worse every time," Ten-Trees said, approaching the soaked man. "How can people live like this?"

"Careful," I cautioned, twisting the water handle closed. "He's holding his arm funny. It might be broken."

Ten-Trees nodded and gingerly touched John Doe on the opposite shoulder.

"NIGGER! FAGGOT! LIAR!" John Doe thundered, suddenly energized beyond anything you would expect from his scrawny, malnourished frame. He attacked Ten-Trees, pummeling his broad back with a rain of wild, whirling blows.

"FUCKING FAGGOT SPIES!!" he screamed as Ten-Trees covered his face. Bull and I each grabbed one flailing arm while Ten-Trees corralled both kicking legs. Bumping and jostling, we fell into a dripping, feces-splattered pile. It took us more than a minute to finally pin our patient to the asphalt.

"FAGGOTS! NIGGERS!" John Doe shrieked attempting to wriggle free, but he was at last secure. The back ER door opened. Maria Gonzales, a nurse, surveyed the situation. "Can't you boys play nice?" she said with a smile.

"Call security," Bull said, struggling to suppress one last fling of the man's extremity.

"Done," Maria replied and closed the door.

Bull, Ten-Trees and I, still puffing, eyed each other. We were hot, wet and streaked with things none of us wanted to identify.

"Vitamin H?" Ten-Trees asked while we waited for help. He was referring to Haldol, a powerful anti-psychotic medication.

"Five milligrams IM," I agreed. "With one of Cogentin and two of Ativan."

Haldol would, hopefully, put John Doe out for a few hours. Cogentin is used to combat a side effect of Haldol, painful muscle cramps called "dystonias." Ativan is like a quick acting Valium. It helps quiet any situation. This Haldol, Cogentin and Ativan combination, given by injection, is the standard psych ER cocktail for violent psychotic episodes. It's enough medication to drop a horse.

Finally, three burly security guards arrived and, after a bit more scuffling, escorted our equally winded patient back into the ER and to a restraint room. There he would be sedated, get some sleep, be given a decent shower and a good looking over. Watching John Doe depart, I felt something in my hair. Reaching up, I pulled out two squirming lice and, without a thought, snapped them dead between my thumbnails.

I returned to the nursing station, washed my hands then spotted the two cops just finishing their part of John Doe's paperwork, a detailed legal document called a "72 Hour Hold" or "5150" as it's known in our business. The term 5150 refers to the section in California's Welfare and Institutions Code that allows for a mentally ill person's detainment.

With so many homeless, psychotic people living in the streets, policemen write a lot of 5150s. They don't like it, and I don't blame them. It takes up an inordinate amount of time.

"What's the point of this?" the first cop said to his partner, tapping the 5150 with a pen. They didn't know I was standing behind them. "We pick up the same miserable people over and over and they end up back on the street a week later. I'm beginning to spend more time in this damn psych hospital than I do on patrol. I know the local crazies better than the criminals."

"They should just declare mental illness illegal," he went on. "Hell, it's easier and more humane to arrest them."

Unfortunately, he was right. The largest population of seriously mentally ill people in the United States is in the LA county jail, not because they've committed a major crime but, something to which the cop had eluded, eventually there's nothing else to do with them.

"What a fuckin' mess," he added.

The other cop shook his head. "It's the way things are. Who knows why?"

I walked up to the pair and took the 5150 from them. "Thanks," I said.

The first cop was still irritated. "What kind of system is this anyway? We've got better things to do than haul around all the nuts you keep letting loose. Can't you get these people off the street? Aren't there clinics or something?"

"There used to be," I said. "And state hospitals, too."

"Somebody sure fucked things up."

"It would seem so."

The second cop checked his belt, gun and pockets. "Gotta go," he said, gently pushing his partner. He turned to me as they left the psych ER. "Forgive him. He's new."

"Me too," I said behind them as the exit door swung closed.

Although in my forties, I'd only recently become a psychiatrist. It's different than most people think. It's different than I had thought it was going to be.

II

I didn't get involved with this slime and insanity business on purpose. I had something else in mind entirely. I came to psychiatry in mid-career after a painfully gruesome nine years as an emergency room physician, like you see on TV in *ER*. My partners and I ran a level-one trauma center in a large southwestern city. During that span I'd seen misery, death, violence and deprivation in every conceivable form. Or so I thought.

In the ER I was so constantly covered with blood that at the end of each day, I used a toothpick to clean it from the rims of my glasses. It became routine. Like brushing my teeth.

Then, events began to unravel. I began to unravel. One night we had to resuscitate four shooting victims all of whom were bleeding to death at the same time. Unfortunately, there were only three breathing tubes. Someone had to go. I did a quick ID check and selected the oldest. We worked on the other three as a middle-aged man died quietly, alone, his life oozing onto the tile floor unattended.

As it turned out, my final day in the ER went similarly: a huge multi-car pile up on the freeway, too many patients all at once, too much blood, not enough nurses, equipment or medication. Our trauma team was trying to save a phalanx of battered people who, it seemed, wouldn't stop coming. After what felt like an eternity, it was finally over.

When the carnage had been sorted, as the floors were being mopped, I glanced up from a mountain of paperwork into one of our three previously teeming trauma rooms. There, amid a jungle of IV tubes hanging from the ceiling, heaps of broken medicine ampoules on the floor and scores of wet X-rays thrown helter-skelter onto still-lit viewers on the wall, was the body of a little girl. She lay on a stretcher that had been inadvertently pushed to the back of the room, patiently waiting her turn to be treated, her turn to be saved. But, somehow in all the din and confusion, we'd forgotten about her. Lying face up, one arm dangling slightly to the side, she was, of course, long since dead.

Staring at her thin, lifeless body, I knew it was over. The next morning I called and said I wouldn't be coming to work that day or ever again. I was a wreck. Something major had to change. I had to start over.

After a few weeks of thought, psychiatry seemed like a quiet respite from the ER's constant chaos. Frankly, I didn't know much about the field; during medical school I'd spent four weeks working at an outpatient clinic and had attended the mandatory eight lectures. I pictured myself in a spacious office nodding occasionally and saying "Hmmm...Tell me more."

With a renewed sense of purpose, I applied for and was accepted into a psychiatric residency training program at a Southern California county hospital, which I completed four years later. During that time, I first learned how hard psychiatrists work. I'd honestly thought and wondered out loud to my wife what could a psychiatrist possibly do during training that would take four years? And especially on call at night, keeping watch over the ward patients, surely it meant nothing more than settling in front of a TV and answering the occasional phone call. My first night in the hospital I admitted eleven patients through the psych ER, each more crazy and violent than the next. There were constant medication decisions, blood work to interpret, people to wrestle into restraints, men with chest pain, pregnant women beginning labor. Drugs. Voices. Screaming. When I drove home the next afternoon I fell asleep behind the wheel of my car in the driveway. It never got any easier.

Now I'm a psychiatrist at another large county hospital in Los Angeles. Its official name is the Benjamin H. Miller Medical Center. On the street it's known simply as the "Mill," an enormous medical complex of which the hospital is only one part. There are outpatient offices, research buildings, large bungalows for vehicle storage and huge mechanical sheds constantly billowing steam as they supply power and heat to all the surrounding structures. There are cafeterias, laboratories, a helicopter landing pad, waiting rooms, sidewalks, parking lots and gift shops, all the services necessary for an enclosed community—which is what the Mill really is. The place encompasses four square blocks.

In the northeast corner of this city-within-a-city is the eight-story hospital proper, the heart of the medical center. This is where the action is, where life wrestles with death on a daily basis.

Being a county-run, public facility, the Mill cares for the people in our section of LA who have no money, no insurance, no place else to go. It's the last stop on the medical train. If we can't save you, you won't get saved.

Our hospital is what's known as a "teaching" institution. We train newly graduated doctors to become specialists in their chosen fields. They get to learn from, or "practice" on, if you will, the indigent citizens of LA County. The young doctors are known as the "housestaff" or, more specifically, "interns" during their first year and "residents" for three years thereafter. All housestaff are under the supervision of staff doctors called "attendings" of which I'm one.

Every medical service is available at the Mill, almost always in state-of-the-art form. Teaching institutions are, by and large, the finest hospitals in the country.

At the Mill, the in-patient psychiatry ward occupies half of the sixth floor. Other floors are filled with patients from surgery, general medicine, gynecology, cardiology, etc. The operating rooms are on the second story of the building. There are four separate emergency rooms, medical (for heart attacks, trauma and the like), obstetric, pediatric and psychiatric, all at ground level. The psych ER is where I met John Doe.

I have two jobs at the Mill. I'm what's called a "ward chief," which means I'm one of the doctors ultimately responsible for what happens to our hospitalized patients. I also run the psych ER on specified days, seeing people as they come in off the street, many of whom get transferred up to the ward.

For that year, Drs. Yang and Dupree were my housestaff. They would go where I went, do what I did, being taught as I'd been taught. Their time with me would be a learning experience. As it turned out, I would learn the most of all.

III

After our battle with John Doe, the rest of the day proceeded apace—one human disaster after another. By 4:30 we were exhausted. Fortunately, it was time for the twice-daily ritual known as "sign-out" rounds, a detailed explanation to the on-coming night shift, who would staff the ER until morning, of our remaining patients and their problems. Next time, the staff would sign out the old patients, and anyone newly admitted during the night, back to us again.

In charge of the night doctors was DuBerry "Bear" Boudreaux, a hulking, ghetto-razored, genius of a man. An area icon, I'd known Bear since my days as a resident. I admired him as much as anyone I'd ever known. He'd been raised in the sinkhole neighborhood our hospital served, overcoming the gangs, poverty and violence to obtain a Harvard education, both undergraduate and medical school. Then, to his credit, with job offers from every conceivable source, he'd returned home to serve those around whom he'd grown up.

The fact that Bear was blind made his accomplishments even more amazing. His attendant sunglasses only added to an already substantial presence. Picture Ray Charles in a linebacker's body, and you had Bear.

I'd worked with Bear just over a year but we weren't close. He let few people into his inner world and I, as yet, wasn't one. For instance, I didn't know how he'd lost his sight. There'd just never seemed a good time to ask.

Bear eased into a chair in the doctors lounge, a small room off the ER nursing station. I sat opposite him in a casual circle. Yang and Dupree, worn out from the day, slumped in their seats, lazily thumbing through small packets of index cards that contained all the information, in condensed form, on their patients. They'd both learned, as I had during my training, that you can't keep age, sex, family history, medications, recent events and a myriad collection of laboratory data for fifteen patients in your head, so they used note cards. Almost all doctors-in-training do this.

The rest of the night crew came through the door. If the day group was tired, the night people looked even worse. Dr. Mary Redmond, generally a cheery, brash Texan, was sullen and moody. Her partner, Dr. Nick Hundley, a somewhat dour New Yorker, was almost catatonic. Tina Jacobs, a pixie-cute, blonde medical student from UCLA, completed the list. Tina had been assigned to Bear's night shift with Redmond and Hundley for the past week but was coming to join Yang, Dupree and me on Monday. "Nice woman, very bright," Bear had said about her. "But not much interested in psychiatry."

The reason for the on-coming housestaff's depressed state was that, as a requirement of their training, they were mandated to do "night call." This meant running the psych ER and keeping an eye on our ward patients every fourth night, in addition to working somewhere else in the hospital all day. For our young doctors it was psychosis, body secretions, medication decisions and crisis for thirty-six hours straight. I'd done the same thing during my residency. It damn near killed me.

Sign-out rounds went quickly. In order, all the ER patients were discussed briefly, a tentative plan of care proposed and any potential problems flagged.

"Springer, Joanne," Yang said. "Twenty-eight-year-old Caucasian female. Tore apart a liquor store. Thought demons were transmitting messages through the bottles. We got a dose of medicine in her. She's sleeping."

"Tox screen?" Bear asked. He had an unerring nose for street drug use.

"Positive for speed," Yang replied. "She'll probably clear up. Leave her. I'll boot her out in the morning."

In addition to being the homeless, psychotic, street person capital of the world, Southern California is the amphetamine epicenter as well. It makes for an ugly mix.

"Taofa, Manu, thirty-nine-year-old Samoan male," Dupree continued. "Whacked his parents with a baseball bat then trashed the house. Voices told him to do it. He's in restraints. Took five cops to put him down. Got some Haldol. He's snoozing too." She brushed a wisp of hair away from her forehead. "Chronic schizophrenic. He'll need to come in. Our beds are full, maybe something will break tomorrow."

Bear shook his head. "How badly were his folks beaten?"

"Mom's upstairs on the third floor," Dupree replied. "Broken ribs. Compound fracture of the femur."

And so it went. A gruesome recitation was given of half-naked women found wandering in traffic, unbathed men discovered in sewers, IV drugs, AIDS, voices, delusions, slashed wrists, until we'd finished with all fourteen patients save one.

"John Doe," Yang said. In all his visits, he'd never given us a name or any other information for that matter. "Found walking down the freeway. S.O.S. Same old shit."

"Again?" Bear murmured.

"I dug out his file." Yang continued. "Eighty-four hospital admits in the past four years."

Up to that point quiet and unassuming, Tina showed some spark. "That's ridiculous," she said, her eyes flashing. Then she caught herself. "Sorry. No offense."

"None taken," I replied and meant it.

After rounds, as I was preparing to go home, Tina motioned me toward the other side of the nursing station.

"Could I interview John Doe?" she asked unexpectedly.

"Of course. I'll sit in with you."

I retrieved the man from his room. He looked much better after a long shower, an industrial strength delousing and a heavy dose of medication. He almost seemed normal, if you ignored rotting teeth, the missing parts of three fingers and a festering wound near his right shoulder. Despite the scouring and a clean hospital gown, a strong hint of his previous smell still lingered. I took he and Tina into a small interview room.

Once inside, Tina sat to my left with John Doe on my right. She smiled, clicking a pen over a blank pad of paper. "You're listed as John Doe," she said professionally. "What's your real name?"

No sooner were the words out of her mouth than John Doe went off like a rocket.

"YOU LYING NAZI CUNT!!!" he screamed and came at Tina with fists clenched. I lunged forward, deflecting his initial punch. We tumbled to the floor, chairs flying. And for the second time that day, John Doe and I grappled.

Fortunately, Bull was soon at the door with Yang and Hundley in tow. Between the four of us we managed to again subdue our patient, holding him until the security police arrived. It was the same group who'd responded to the previous call. As they trundled John Doe back to his room, one of the officers shot a glance over his shoulder that said, "How stupid do you have to be?"

When Bear finally appeared, Yang, Hundley, Bull and I were just getting off the linoleum. Tina hadn't moved an inch. Her pen was still poised. Eyes big as dinner plates, her mouth was agape.

"Everybody all right?" Bear asked, his hand on the door frame.

"Yeah, we're fine, Bear," I said.

"Good God," Tina finally sighed. She'd returned to the planet.

Trying to catch my breath, I bent at the waist, put both hands on my knees and lowered my head.

"You're lucky he didn't kill you both," Yang whispered, equally spent. I didn't reply.

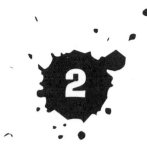

2 Serpents and Psychosis

WHEN I FINALLY LEFT THE PSYCH ER, I WAS DRAINED. At least it was Friday and, except for the occasional phone call, this meant a two-day respite from the tumult at work. The hospital chaos continued on during the weekend, of course, but everything was handled by the interns and residents. Their hellish week not being enough, they rotated twenty-four-hour shifts on Saturday and Sunday as well. I was available but only by beeper. For attendings, this is what is known as being "on call." If a serious emergency arose, I would go to the hospital, but in psychiatry that doesn't happen often.

Driving home that evening, however, wasn't the relieved pleasure it should have been. I knew the upcoming days would be tense. Of late things at the Seager house hadn't been going well.

My wife Linda was anxious and not hiding it very successfully. Her mood was beginning to make the kids nervous, too. Even the family cat, Lasorda—named after the portly Dodger manager—was starting to act funny.

Linda's emotional state could best be summarized by "The Look." The Look was hard to describe exactly, but it seemed to be a combination of anger and resentment tinged with a veneer of hurt. It was guaranteed to generate in me the maximum amount of guilt possible. Nothing made me feel worse than The Look.

It had taken me a while to realize that Linda's expression was a variation of one my mother had occasionally used on me as a child. The message was clear: "You let me down."

I was getting The Look a lot lately and knew why. It had initially appeared when, toward the end of my residency, I'd mentioned the possibility of my working full-time at the Mill. I'd just spent four years of psychiatric training at another county hospital, a bizarre, impossible place, ensconced in the most cancerous neighborhood of LA. I'd learned a lot there, mainly what it meant to be a modern psychiatrist.

Linda understood this. For those four years she'd tolerated my mood swings, lack of sleep and periods of obsessive study without a whimper. "It's knowing that you're driving into that damn ghetto every day that kills me," she said once without being asked. Apparently she'd suffered more than I realized.

Linda's only comfort had been the knowledge that my training would one day come to an end. That I'd finally take a real job with real hours for real pay. The ghetto and public sector psychiatry would soon be a thing of the past. Then I brought up the Mill. That's when I first got The Look.

So what made me do what I did? What made me even consider working at the Mill after four long years at County General? What was the real reason I took another public job, treating the sickest-of-the-sick, known in the vernacular as "train wrecks"?

There was something, I concluded, that excited me about a sick soul, abandoned by society and God, coming in from the fog. Seeing John Doe cleaned up and seeming human again reminded me of all the scrambled, crusted people the police had hauled in over the past few years. They looked so much better after such simple actions as removing their rags, taking a bath and eating a few good meals.

Given the correct anti-psychotic medication, almost everyone improved and some remarkably so. It was an amazingly gratifying experience, as much as any satisfaction I'd had in other branches of medicine. As a psychiatrist, I felt more like a doctor than at any time in my life.

Simultaneously, however, I realized there was clearly an aspect of psychiatry that wasn't right. An uneasiness began to grow during my residency, but then I'd been too busy reading and trying to survive the brutal schedule to sort things out. John Doe's arrival in the ER, however, had rekindled my budding confusion. We had good medications, competent doctors, accurate diagnoses, yet our patients still looked worse each time we saw them. Regardless of what we did, no matter how much better they got in the hospital, this never seemed to change. Eighty-four hospital visits by one person in four years didn't make sense to me. Something was wrong.

I tried not to let these ruminations interfere with my time off. Linda and I kept a respectful tone to our conversation, and it was great spending time with the kids. Nevertheless, I was disconcerted, and she was angry. Events were coming to a head.

On Sunday night, I drifted off to sleep thinking of John Doe.

II

The next Monday I wasn't feeling much better. I arrived at the Mill and, as usual, went to my office first. It was down a short corridor just off the psych ER lobby, a room crowded with folding chairs where people who'd walked in off the street were waiting to be seen. It was 8:00 A.M., and already the place was nearly full.

When I got to my office door, Tina was there. Apparently she'd been thinking about John Doe as well. She had a psychiatric text under each arm. There was a pile of medical journals at her feet.

"Hello," I said, sliding a key into the door and swinging it open. "Anything left in the library?"

Tina gathered the magazines and blew into the room, hurriedly dumping her stack of material onto a clear spot atop my cluttered desk and pulling up a chair.

"Come in," I said, smiling to myself and walking in to join her.

My office was small, which made for unintentional intimacy. There was room for a county-issue metal desk, two utilitarian wooden chairs and a bookcase, the main purpose of which was to store an occasional sack lunch. The only concession I'd made to decor were two posters pinned to the far wall. One was of an alpine vista, probably Switzerland, the other was an action shot of Kenny "The Snake" Stabler during his quarterback days for the old Oakland Raiders. The landscape had been there when I arrived. I'd hung the football shot.

In a break with tradition, there weren't any framed diplomas around, a practice that had always struck me as marginally ostentatious. Besides, we'd moved over the summer and I wasn't entirely certain where mine were anyway. So, beneath the scenes of intense gridiron action and pristine, snow-capped peaks, I sat behind my desk and turned toward Tina.

"I'm guessing this has to do with John Doe."

"Of course," Tina replied with uncharacteristic verve. "But not just him. It's this whole business of schizophrenia. I spent most of the weekend reading. It's such an interesting disease."

"Interesting?" I'd always struggled with a tragic illness being called "interesting" or "fascinating"; it seemed to ignore the pain involved. Yet, doctors do this a lot.

"I never knew it was such a complex mix of sophisticated neuro-chemistry, genetics, social factors and history," Tina went on rapidly. "There's so much more to these people than I'd imagined."

Tina's sudden enthusiasm was something new, and I wanted to encourage it. For the next hour, we discussed the various brain structure and cerebral chemical abnormalities thought to be central to schizophrenia.

One theory states that the disease is caused by an alteration in dopamine function, a prominent neurotransmitter. In some schizophrenics, the molecule seems to function at abnormally high levels. Most anti-psychotic drugs block the action of dopamine and, as such, decrease the psychosis and disordered thinking so prevalent in the disorder.

Others believe that schizophrenia results from an in-utero infection. More schizophrenics are born in the winter when viral disease is most common. A few scientists feel phencyclidine, the street drug PCP, may be to blame. Amazingly, your brain produces this chemical naturally and, perhaps, the thinking goes, it might be acting at excessive levels in schizophrenics.

Most likely, however, schizophrenia is a developmental disorder, an unnatural disruption in the way your brain is wired from birth, resembling more a form of dementia or brain failure. Once it sets in, those afflicted tend to have a drop in IQ scores averaging about forty-five points. Luckily, newly discovered but surprisingly old-and-ignored evidence suggests that the disease process may be interrupted or halted by early intervention.

As we talked, Tina's enthusiasm increased. "I didn't know these people could do so well," she said almost indignantly. "Seven out of ten respond to medication. That's phenomenal."

"You're right."

"Think of the difference it could make to John Doe," Tina continued. "He might come in from Outer Space permanently."

"If we can persuade him to take it."

Tina looked puzzled. "Why wouldn't he? Who'd want to hurt like that?"

"Schizophrenia and medication is a touchy subject," I replied.

"Touchy?" Tina stammered. "It seems pretty clear to me."

I glanced at my watch. The story of medication and schizophrenia would have to wait. "Let's head up to the ward. We're late for rounds."

Tina stood. "Can we talk again?"

"Anytime."

"Tomorrow then, if that's alright?" she said. "So much suffering doesn't make sense. I'm confused."

Tina's sense of frustration about schizophrenia and its treatment was understandable. The disease has confounded science

for millennia. The discovery of the first useful drugs was long and circuitous; one medicine was produced from a nineteenth century cloth dye and another, a root, had been underfoot unrecognized for thousands of years.

III

In 1573, botanist Leonard Rauwolf was dispatched from England to explore and catalogue the pharmaceutical plants of the Orient. Among other flora, he took special interest in a shrub known by its Hindu name "Pagla-ka-dawa" or the "insanity herb." An extract of its root was reputed to be a cure for snakebite, cataracts, cholera and psychosis, as evidenced by extensive descriptions of the potion's uses in ancient Ayurvedic Hindu medical texts. The active chemical was eventually isolated and named Rauwolfia Serpentina. Later it acquired the generic name "reserpine."

Despite the age-old claim that the drug could cure madness, the compound's effect on mental illness wasn't tested until 1931 when two Indian physicians, Sen and Bose, finally administered it to a group of schizophrenic patients. Remarkably, it worked. Equally as surprising, this achievement was ignored for another twenty years. In 1953, a second pair of Indian doctors, Hakim and Ahmabad, reported that reserpine's use on schizophrenics produced a fifty-one percent recovery rate.

This result finally caught people's attention. Dr. Nathan Kline, research director at Rockland State Hospital in New York, introduced reserpine to the United States. He gave the preparation to two hundred "severely disturbed" institutionalized schizophrenic patients, twenty-two percent of which improved enough to be discharged.

After thousands of years of trial and error (a subject we'll address later), at last a medication had been proven effective in treating schizophrenic psychosis. The age-old barrier was finally broken. But was it the best drug? Were there others? That answer would come from a German textile chemist named Bernthsen, searching for an improved method of coloring his cloth.

In 1890, Bernthsen concocted a new class of thread dyes called phenothiazines. Later, biologist Paul Ehrlich discovered that one of the phenothiazines, methelene blue, was toxic to insect larvae and swine parasites. In the 1940s these compounds were sprayed in African swamps to kill malaria-carrying mosquitoes.

To understand how an insecticide could become a psychiatric medicine, we have to explain the phenothiazines' connection to histamine, the body chemical that makes you sneeze. During the early 1950s, histamine was found to be the agent responsible for human allergic reactions. Soon after, Daniel Bouer, a researcher at the Pasteur Institute in Paris, theorized that histamine blockers, or "antihistamines," must also exist. He began to search for this hypothetical

substance and some of the chemicals tested were Bernthsen's phenothiazines. Amazingly, these cloth-dye/insect-poisons proved to
be just what he was looking for. They did block the effects of histamine. This led to the production of a phenothiazine derivative, di-
phenhydramine (Benedryl), the drug currently employed in a
number of cold and allergy medications.

At the same time, another phenothiazine, promazine, was created in France. As often happens with a new discovery, chemists began tinkering with its structure. When a chlorine molecule was added
to the promazine framework, it became chlorpromazine and was
given the trade name of Thorazine.

Thorazine, as do all phenothiazines, also contains anti-
histaminic properties. Its first use, however, was not as an allergy
medication but as an adjunctive medium for surgical anesthesia.

In experiments aimed at combating a potentially lethal low blood
pressure state common to anesthetics of the time, Henri Laborit, a
Paris surgeon, tried giving Thorazine to his patients prior to operating
on them. His hunch was this: the blood pressure problem associated
with general anesthesia was related to the body's release of histamine, and Thorazine might combat it. He was correct. This discovery was credited with saving the lives of thousands of wounded
French soldiers requiring surgery during the Indochina war.

Laborit also made another significant observation. In addition to
stopping surgical low blood pressure, Thorazine made his patients
unusually calm. They were tranquil but not drowsy. He passed this
information on to his psychiatric colleagues at St. Anne's Hospital in
Paris.

At Laborit's urging, Jean Delay and Pierre Deniker began using
Thorazine as a treatment for the psychosis and agitation associated
with schizophrenia. Their results were dramatic and soon this new
"anti-psychotic" medication was in use across Europe.

The first American trial of Thorazine occurred in 1954. It was
given to all of one state hospital's supposedly "incurable" schizophrenics, and twenty-five percent were able to be discharged. More
research ensued. Kris tracked three hundred formerly institutionalized patients treated with Thorazine and found that, if they contin-

ued to take their medication, sixty-three percent had not required rehospitalization after five years of follow-up.

Thus, by the mid-twentieth century, there were two medications, Thorazine and reserpine, which could safely and easily treat psychosis. Eventually, Thorazine was found to be more effective and to cause fewer side effects. Other classes of drugs were soon developed that had properties similar to Thorazine. Notably, in 1959, Paul Janssen, while experimenting with Demerol derivatives in search of a new pain killer, synthesized Haldol which remains to this day a mainstay in anti-psychotic drug therapy.

As the 1960s dawned, the treatment of mental illness, and specifically the psychosis associated with schizophrenia, seemed to be on the verge of a golden age. Management of this dreaded disease would be specific and accurate. The lives of the severely mentally ill were destined to improve dramatically. Unfortunately, even with the advent in the past three decades of even better anti-psychotic drugs, this promise of a better future never materialized. In fact, as it turned out, the only verge the mentally ill were upon was the verge of cataclysm.

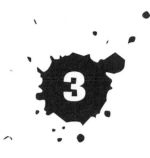

The Tower of Babble

AFTER OUR INITIAL CONVERSATION, Tina and I began to meet for an hour each day, as schedules allowed. Standard practice in psychiatry between an attending and student, it's called "supervision." We discussed the diagnosis and treatment of the serious mental disorders from which our patients suffered, usually bipolar disorder, major depression and schizophrenia.

We talked specifically about John Doe. After he was sent up from the ER to the in-patient ward, I assigned him to Tina's care. During those first few days, we also spoke about ourselves. It was a chance for me to get to know Tina.

She was from Chicago. I'm a serious baseball fan so naturally my first question was "Sox or Cubs?" Her answer: "You a National or American League man?"

Being a Dodger fan that one was easy. "National League."

"Love those Cubs," Tina replied diplomatically. "As Ernie Banks said, 'Let's play two.'"

Tina was the youngest of three children. Her father had been a physician, a fairly renowned surgeon on the North Side, which helped explain her initial indifference toward psychiatry. Surgeons and psychiatrists are the medical world's equivalent of cobras and mongooses, real "oil and water" stuff. Surgeons consider us to be prattling chatterers. Psychiatrists feel most of them are obsessive robots. Suffice it to say, there's built-in friction.

Tina's father had passed away when she was twelve. "Cancer," she said with a tear. "Can you believe it? That was his specialty."

Tina spoke lovingly of a sister, an attorney, who lived in New York. But that was nothing compared to the feelings she expressed for her older brother. "He got lost for a while in the sixties," she said. "But he came around. Graduated first in his class at Yale Medical. I think he's the best person I know." Her eyes were glowing.

"Surgeon?"

"Of course."

Tina was a little older than the average medical student of her station, something I'd noted occurring with greater frequency of late. Medical school, for Tina's generation, was much more of a real occupational choice than the often life-and-death decision it had been for my group. We'd had students come through the Mill who'd gone to dental school for a while, surfed in Hawaii or played piano in a cocktail lounge after college. I'd applied to medical school during the Vietnam War. My options had been simpler. I either began studying cadavers or risked becoming one.

The best part of Tina and my talks, however, were our discussions about John Doe. Early on I'd cautioned her about what psychiatrists call a "rescue fantasy" which is wanting so much for someone to get better that you don't see things logically. You invest enormous amounts of energy toward saving a patient who cannot or does not want to be saved. This effort says more about the doctor than the patient.

I had a hard time giving Tina my rescue fantasy speech because as she continued to work closely with John Doe, the man truly was being saved. He was taking his anti-psychotic medication on a regular basis and had stopped acting like someone from Mars. He'd even become civil.

Nonetheless, I was familiar with public sector psychiatry and knew how capricious a patient's choice to take medicine could be. As well, the Superior Court was about to become involved in John Doe's case. Following a number of judicial rulings over the past twenty-five years, judges or their designees make many decisions about our patients' care—not doctors. One of those determinations, whether a patient can remain hospitalized against his will and continue to receive psychiatric care, is the initial issue upon which they rule.

John Doe's first hearing was coming soon. I didn't have the heart to tell Tina what was probably going to happen.

II

Three times a week the in-patient staff meets for a ritual known as "ward rounds." Rounds are when the entire treatment team—doctors, nurses, social workers, psychologists and students—gather in a conference room around a large table to discuss each patient in detail in order to outline care options, make medication decisions and develop discharge plans. It's an hour spent making certain we're all on the same page. We convened at 9:00 A.M. every Monday, Wednesday and Friday.

That Wednesday morning, after a short visit to my office, I headed up the elevator to the sixth floor. Unlocking the large metal ward door with its small wire-reinforced window, I walked inside.

There are twenty-four beds on the in-patient unit. They're grouped into a section of rooms with either four or two beds or a single bed. The latter are reserved for the more actively psychotic or obstreperous patients. All the rooms fan off a single hallway that runs in a big horseshoe around that half of the building. A cafeteria where the patients take their hospital-kitchen-prepared meals, is at the end of the hall on the closed part of the horseshoe. Beside it is a recreation or "day room" filled with games, a piano and a pool table. The conference room is just around the bend. The far corridor contains offices. Each member of the housestaff has one, as does the head nurse, our psychologist and social worker.

A glassed-in nurses station is about three-quarters of the way down the first leg of the hallway. That's where the patients' charts, medications and paperwork are kept. As well, there's counter space and room for five or six people to sit. It's where "progress notes," the doctor's daily, written record of his patients' condition, and "orders"—requests for the lab to draw blood tests or for radiology to do X-rays, etc.—are written in the charts. If time warrants, the nursing station is also where the staff converges for conversation.

Walking toward the conference room, I passed a dozen people ambling, shuffling or just standing in the hallway. I heard Japanese, Korean, Spanish and Chinese being spoken. Other weeks it would be Vietnamese, Lao, Hindi and Tagalog. I said hello to each person going by and, in true LA style, got most of my replies in some language other than English. As LA has grown into a polyglot of immigrant nationalities, so has our patient population.

Imagine the difficulty in determining what makes sense and what doesn't from a patient speaking only a regional Peruvian Indian dialect? Our ward had become a sort of United Nations of the Insane, a true Tower of Babel, the inhabitants of which were, unfortunately, babbling.

An extreme example of what can happen in this situation occurred a few months ago. A Pakistani patient came to the ward and only spoke Urdu. To converse with him I had to recruit an array of people. The patient's brother spoke Urdu but also Hindi. A cousin spoke Hindi but not Urdu and, miraculously, some Spanish as well. I called Maria from the Psych ER to translate the Spanish to me. We stood in a line, me at one end, the patient at the other. I asked a question, and it got passed down from person to person; the reply arrived in the same way. The process more resembled a bucket brigade or party game than medicine. I finally gave up when I asked "Are you hearing voices?" and the daisy chain translation came back "June fourteenth."

Near the conference room door, I met John Doe. "Hello," he said. As I passed, he whispered, "Nazi." I turned, but he didn't look back.

"Good morning, girlfriend," Yang said as I walked in. It was his standard greeting. Yang was gay but never so openly as when he was around the ward's head nurse Phyllis Yates. Yang liked to needle her every chance he got. Evangelical by nature, she thought Yang was a crime against Nature.

"Good morning, dear," I replied, ruffling Yang's hair. Yates visibly stiffened. I liked to pull her chain a bit, too.

The rest of the staff quickly assembled. To my right was Carol Nguyen, a petite Asian nurse. Next was Paul Salazar, a modest, immensely compassionate social worker. Salazar was gold to us. Raised in southern Texas, he spoke fluent Spanish. Then came Yang and Dupree, an elegant, aristocratic black woman from Georgia, by way of Princeton. Dupree could have been a runway model but had found her way into psychiatry instead.

Across the table was Nancy Hopkins, a sturdy, reliable nurse, Nicolette "Nicki" Larson, a nursing aide, and Evelyn Townes, the ward psychologist. Townes and I had connected the moment we met. She also had two sons involved in baseball and a husband as possessed by the sport as I. Finally, Tina entered the room behind me.

Rounds went quickly. Yang or Dupree began with a capsulized recitation of each patient's history, explaining the string of terrible events which had led to their being hospitalized, and ending with a summary of everyone's individualized medication regimen. The nurses followed with their report—were our patients eating, dressing themselves, bathing, conversing?—things we all take for granted but which become deeply disrupted when serious mental illness strikes.

Finally, Salazar detailed the discharge plans. This was where the system began to break down. We knew what was probably best for our patients once they left the ward, what would maximize their well-being and eventual return to health—a safe place to live, regular doctor visits and continued medication. But either these things weren't available (LA County had suffered a series of severe mental health budget cuts, which had closed most outpatient clinics), the patients' often didn't want them or, astonishingly, the court wouldn't allow it.

I felt sorry for Salazar. I had no idea how he avoided the resignation typical of people in his position. Despite the difficulties, he kept plugging away. He continually struggled to find facilities which would give our patients follow-up appointments that, for reasons I'll explain later, they rarely kept. He placed them in board-and-care homes from which they would routinely walk away. He made certain I wrote prescriptions; many, we knew, would go unfilled.

"How do you do it?" I asked him once. "What keeps you going?"

Salazar's usual smile vanished. "The system is screwed up," he said. "Our patients are suffering. But I do what I can. One thought gives me hope. When things finally do change for the better, and they will, I want to be there. I want to be part of doing it right for once."

"And this sustains you?" I asked, impressed as always by the man's genuine decency.

"That," Salazar replied with a wink. "And Prozac helps a lot, too."

III

I run a loose ship during rounds. There is always time for a joke, a story, pictures of a wedding or someone's kids. Yates had intimated that my approach was somewhat less than professional, that more medical formality was in order, that letting Yang recite a bawdy limerick showed a lack of concern for our patients and respect for the staff. Yates and I had gotten off on the wrong foot. My first day on the ward, at the beginning of rounds, she'd asked me what I preferred to be called. "You can call me Steve," I said. "Or Doctor Seager. Or what my wife calls me when we have a fight—'Mr. Big-Fuckin'-Know-It-All-Psychiatrist.'" Everyone laughed except Yates. I was a bit of a flake, she was something of a priss, but over the years we'd learned to get along.

I had chosen my administrative style on purpose. There's only so much tragedy a person can handle, and our chronically mentally ill patients were just that—tragedies. Dealing with the results of long-standing disease and neglect was difficult. I knew it was better to let the staff blow off some steam than blow apart.

During rounds, the final detail to be discussed was each patient's legal status. This meant determining where they stood in the labyrinthine, contradictory maze of judicial rights versus treatment issues, a recitation of how close they were to being dumped into the streets again.

"John Doe," Yates said.

Tina sat up straight. "John Doe is a young Caucasian male with eighty-four hospital admissions in the last four years. His place of birth is uncertain. No information available about his childhood. Family history is unknown. His problems seem to have begun..."

"Cut to the chase," Yang interjected. "You can write his biography in the chart."

While detailed information about each patient's history was important, we were too busy during rounds for frills. The residents had the patter down cold. What's the problem and how do we solve it? It's a side effect of working in a system overloaded with incredibly sick people and not enough staff.

"Don't worry, every new student does it. You'll learn," Yang said with a smile. "The facts ma'am, just the facts," he added in his best Joe Friday imitation.

"Mr. Doe was found wandering down the 91 freeway covered in feces and flies," Tina began again after a pause. "Keeps mumbling about the FBI and wires. He's been in restraints twice since admission. Threatened to punch the night nurse and got into a scuffle yesterday morning during breakfast. Some argument about a muffin. Called another patient a 'Nazi faggot.'"

"Interesting thought," Yang mused and Yates shot him a glance.

"Orthopedics will be up to see about his arm, and we'll get him to Dental Clinic when he finally settles down," Tina continued. "He's on Haldol—five milligrams twice a day with a half milligram of Cogentin. He's still crazy but doing better."

"PC hearing's this afternoon," Tina concluded. Then she shook her head. "I still don't get all this court stuff. Isn't it obvious how sick he is?"

"That's not the issue, girlfriend," Yang said.

IV

To understand what lay ahead for Tina and I, at John Doe's "PC" or "Probable Cause" hearing, it's important to have a cursory understanding of the American legal system as it relates to the mentally ill. This begins with two theoretical foundations which allow us to hold these people involuntarily.

The first principle, *parens patriae*, harkens back to the days of medieval English kings. It states that the monarch is empowered to look after those in his realm who can't care for themselves. He's to act as a "substitute parent" for the enfeebled, insane or those in dire need.

The second doctrine is called "police powers." Conversely, this grants the government the right to protect society from dangerous individuals, entrusting the authorities to act for the public good. We've adopted these tenets and applied them to civil commitment, i.e., we use them as the basis for confining people against their will who haven't committed a crime.

During previous centuries, and for much of this one, institutionalization of the brain diseased was arranged between a patient's family and his doctor, who would petition a judge for a relative's institutionalization. This led to a series of abuses.

Collusion between husbands and judges concerning their soon-to-be ex-wives often provided grounds for divorce. And, not infrequently, heirs to family riches had elderly parents put away to protect against any squandering of the descendents' estate. Responding to this, in 1969, the California Legislature passed the Lanterman-Petris-Short Act, or "LPS" as it has become known. This served as a "model" law that was soon copied in nearly every other state.

The LPS Act removed the judicial power of commitment. No longer could doctors, spouses or relatives simply appeal to the courts for a person's confinement. It set down strict new standards by which hospitals could detain the mentally ill. If a person is dangerous to himself (suicidal), a danger to others (homicidal) or—and the LPS Act coined this term—"gravely disabled," then a three-day evaluation period is permitted, grave disability being defined as unable to provide for one's own "food, clothing or shelter."

After this initial seventy-two hours, if two separate psychiatric examiners concur, an additional fourteen days of hospitalization is allowed. Following that, the patient must either be discharged or placed on a "conservatorship," which mandates the appointment of a legal guardian and possible remanding of the person to a state mental hospital for a time not exceeding one year.

The three California legislators who penned the LPS act had mentally ill persons' best interests at heart and believed they were correcting a grievous injustice. In reality, passage of the LPS Act helped create a national disgrace, the homeless mentally ill.

The Lanterman-Petris-Short Act did something monumental: it radically changed the way mental illness was allowed to be treated. The emphasis was no longer on curing a disease but, instead, everything now focused on protecting the "freedoms" of the brain diseased. It shifted a medical decision into a civil rights issue. As well, it opened a door for the judicial system to invade the day-to-day practice of psychiatry, which the courts did with relish.

Rulings in other states soon followed. A Wisconsin decision, known as *Lessard v. Schmidt*, held that any commitment, "regardless of therapeutic intent," whether criminal in jail or civil in a mental institution, was still incarceration. The court concluded that such acts were unconstitutional unless mentally sick patients were afforded the same legal rights as prisoners, i.e., writs of *habeas corpus* (literally: produce the body), the right to an immediate formal judicial review of a person's case, and other procedurally mandated hearings along the way.

Lessard, as LPS had been, was imitated nationwide. In a few scrawls of the legal pen, the commitment of the mentally ill was now equated with sentencing to the state penitentiary. A previously medical determination had been "criminalized." No longer were decisions concerning mental illness based upon a need for treatment or other compassionate lines, they were about protecting a person's freedom.

The concept of a mental patient's "right to treatment" also developed around this same time. During the first half of this century, many chronically mentally ill or neurologically degenerated persons were exiled to state hospitals where they were at best ignored and at worst abused. Many went totally uncared for. This detainment without treatment became known as "warehousing." It generated public outrage when, in a series of books, newspaper articles, magazine stories and fledgling television reports, the situation was exposed. Lawsuits were filed.

In the early 1970s, the decision in an Alabama class action suit, *Wyatt v. Stickney*, acknowledged a mental patient's right to treatment, and the judge went on to specify exactly how that court guaranteed care would be provided. In 1975, the U.S. Supreme Court ruled on this same matter in perhaps the most famous mental health case ever, *Donaldson v. O'Connor*. The *O'Connor* decision reaffirmed a mental patient's right to treatment, while at the same time concurring with the *Lessard* concept of using legal criteria, or "due process," to decide confinement issues. The judges didn't stop there, however. They went on to state that no one could be hospitalized involuntarily if that person could "survive" by himself in the community. In their written opinion, the justices used the word three times. Severe mental illness was no longer a reason for involuntary hospitalization, as long as you were "surviving."

The final and most currently troublesome area of court interest in mental health began in 1979. In Massachusetts, a state court held that, although institutionalized patients had a right to treatment, they also had the ability to refuse that treatment. This was further clarified in other state court decisions, namely, *Rennie v. Klein* in New Jersey and *Reise v. St. Mary's* in California.

The reasoning behind some of these decisions went so far as to claim that psychotic individuals had a First Amendment, free speech right to their hallucinatory and delusional thinking and any alteration of same by medication would violate the constitution. As well, the California Supreme Court ruled that past behavior patterns may not be weighed as evidence in any current hearing process. The court stated that to grant an involuntary hold based on dangerousness, the danger must be "imminent," i.e., about to happen right then, and that grave disability criteria must be met at the exact moment the patient appears in court.

This process has led to some unusual situations. Mentally ill people may be involuntarily confined for the purpose of treatment, but they can refuse that same treatment and still remain confined. Ironically, the court can now officially order a new form of warehousing (detainment and treatment refusal although treatment is offered) when this was basically the issue that so appalled everyone to begin with. Also, it has led to this eighty-four-admissions-in-four-years business. Many patients, regardless of how many times they've been brought to the hospital, get just well enough to win a hearing and are repeatedly discharged *ad nauseum.*

In short, hospitalization and treatment of the severely brain diseased is a difficult proposition. Tina was about to discover this.

As two o'clock neared, I did my best to prepare her. I outlined the mechanics of the PC process and what would be discussed. I explained that all hearings are adversarial, that there are two sides and testimony is taken. John Doe would be represented by a "patient's rights advocate," someone provided at County expense to serve as his attorney. The advocate would plead to have him released forthwith. I would argue that John Doe needed his involuntary commitment extended, continuing treatment until he was well. A court-appointed "referee" would decide who'd prevailed.

The issue would be whether John Doe met the legal criteria for ongoing commitment: was he dangerous, could he provide for his own food, clothing and shelter? The fact that he was mentally ill would rarely come up.

At PC hearings one side must show "probable cause" that their view is correct in order to "win." If John Doe and his advocate could prove that he was fifty-one percent capable of caring for himself and not dangerous, he would walk out the door.

At a little past two, Mr. Harvey Wentzler, the superior court referee, a bespeckled, humorless man in an off-the-rack gray suit entered the conference room and sat behind the same table we'd sat at that morning during rounds. He opened a scuffed briefcase and spread some papers before him.

Tina sat next to me on Wentzler's right. To his left was John Doe and his advocate, Marcie Atwater, an attractive brunette. She and I had tangled many times in the past.

Wentzler started by speaking to me. "Tell me the patient's diagnosis and his medications."

"Chronic disorganized schizophrenia," I replied. "He's been ordered Haldol—five milligrams twice a day with a half milligram of Cogentin."

"Is Mr. Doe taking his medicine?" Wentzler began filling out a form in front of him.

"Yes," I replied. Should he change his mind, however, this would lead to another hearing down the road.

Wentzler glanced at his paper and then at me again. "You've marked Mr. Doe as a danger to himself."

"He was walking down the 91 freeway."

Wentzler looked at John Doe. "Do you have any plans to kill yourself?"

"Fuck no," John Doe mumbled. And that was that.

Once more Wentzler peered down. "You marked 'danger to others,' Dr. Seager?"

My heart sinking, I cleared my throat. We were going strictly by the book. Barring a miracle, John Doe would be back in traffic by sunset. "He threatened to punch a nurse and got into a fight with another patient."

Then Atwater struck. "That was two days ago." She knew John Doe's chart by heart. "Both nurses' and doctors' notes for the past thirty-six hours show no evidence of such behavior."

"Do you have plans to hurt anyone, Mr. Doe?" Wentzler asked.

"Fuck no," John Doe said again and Wentzler, unflustered, lined that item off his paper. We were now down to the gravely disabled business.

Wentzler got right to the point. "Dr. Seager, do you believe Mr. Doe's mental illness will prevent him from providing for his own food, clothing and shelter?"

I was struggling to control myself. "He was picked up with shit in his pants. We had to burn his clothes." My voice was rising. "He has nothing. How is he going to eat?"

Atwater again. "While it's true that Mr. Doe has no money, he knows the location of two dumpsters behind reputable restaurants which are a continual source of food."

When John Doe nodded in agreement, Wentzler once more marked his paper. I could see the frustration building in Tina's eyes. Her face started to flush. Apparently, court-approved garbage eating didn't sit well with her.

"And where will you live, Mr. Doe?" Wentzler continued. The proceedings were nearing a close.

"Mr. Doe tells me he resides in an abandoned building on 39th and Crenshaw," Atwater interjected. "It provides adequate shelter."

When Wentzler clicked his pen to cross out this final item, I had to put a hand on Tina's arm to keep her from standing.

Then, just when John Doe was about to be freed from his involuntary hold and returned to the abandoned building and restaurant refuse, the miracle happened. As Atwater leaned over to congratulate him, John Doe slapped her right across the face. "You lying slut!" he roared, storming from the room and running down the hall.

Everything was quiet for a moment. Wentzler was stunned. Atwater looked like she'd been struck by lightning. Tina didn't seem able to make sense of anything.

Personally, I had to admit to mixed feelings. I'd secretly wanted to get back at a patient's rights advocate for years.

Destruction of a Delicate Organ

DESPITE HIS OUTBURST AT THE PC HEARING, which resulted in John Doe's hold being prolonged, the man was gradually getting better. On medication, his thoughts had become more organized. He hadn't called anyone a Nazi cunt for three days. After enough showers, the smell and stain were nearly gone from his skin. With the penicillin he'd been taking since admission, his shoulder infection was clearing up. He'd even let the nurses cut his matted hair. Tina bought him a new blue shirt, which he wore with green hospital scrub pants. John Doe was becoming healthier, and Tina was justifiably proud.

I knew we were approaching another danger point, however. Often when horribly sick patients get partially well, they think they're completely cured and stop taking their anti-psychotic medication. It's human nature. The same thing happens with people who need high blood pressure pills. And who hasn't interrupted a course of antibiotics in midstream once the sore throat and fever abate?

The other problem with John Doe's progress was the ever-present court system. As mentioned, every patient has a right to a writ of *habeas corpus*, the court petition for an immediate formal judicial review of his confinement. Winning a writ hearing, exactly like a PC hearing, means instant release from the hospital. The patient's rights advocates pursue these writs vigorously. So, when our sick people finally begin to come up from the deep, they do two things—stop taking their meds and file a writ.

Writ hearings are conducted in front of a superior court judge in a real courtroom. The hospital is represented by the district attorney, the patient, by the public defender. Whenever a patient files a writ, his case is heard within two working days.

I wasn't surprised, then, as I walked onto the ward a few days after John Doe's PC hearing. "Mr. Doe stopped taking his meds," Yates said.

"And he filed a writ," Tina added. "It's set for Monday morning."

"Damn," I muttered. In some weird way I'd begun to like John Doe. After he'd gotten cleaned up, I realized he was only about twenty-five, the same age as my daughter. She was in nursing school and planning to marry. He was eating from trashcans and facing an early death, abandoned and alone on the street.

II

Severe, chronic schizophrenia, the disease from which John Doe suffered, is the most devastating illness a person can contract that doesn't have the decency to kill you. All other human scourges—plague, AIDS, rabies, cancer, etc.—at least cause death. But not chronic schizophrenia. It tortures you instead. You suffer financial death, employment death, social death and, most sadly, personality and intellectual death. But physical death? No. At least not directly. Schizophrenics do die, but it's usually from something else. They freeze in the sewer, wander into traffic, starve or get murdered.

Schizophrenia has always been with us, as ancient a malady as any known to man. Whether called lunacy, witchcraft, mental disorder or mental illness, schizophrenia is, to use a modern phrase, The Mother of All Brain Disease. It makes you hear voices when no one is speaking or commands you through actors on the television. Special messages come directly from God and Satan. The disease turns grammar into gibberish and logic into chaos. Schizophrenia puts shit in your pants and lice on your skin. It turns the world into a disordered, hellish nightmare, as your basic humanity is slowly sucked from you. In the United States, it's the disease that deposits you on the street to be ignored, ridiculed and abused.

Schizophrenia is an equal opportunity destroyer. One percent of the world's population, irrespective of race, religion, sex or culture, comes down with the disease at some point during its lifetime. There are five billion people on the planet, of which fifty million are schizophrenic or will be. In the United States, there are 270 million people; 2.7 million of us have the disease. There are more schizophrenics in our country than people who suffer from end-stage Alzheimer's and multiple sclerosis combined.

Of all places on earth to have schizophrenia, America is one of the worst. The death rate in the United States for schizophrenics is eight times greater than for non-schizophrenics. For those who live on the street, the chance of being murdered is twenty times higher than "normal." One-third of afflicted women in shelters have been raped, ten times the number for the general population. Ten percent of schizophrenics commit suicide, while fifty percent attempt it. Three-hundred thousand of them will die by their own hand. The most common medical problems associated with schizophrenia are scabies, lice, starvation and major trauma, i.e., broken bones from beatings, knife wounds and bullet holes.

Schizophrenia is a disease of the brain, as heart disease affects your heart and liver disease attacks your liver. You don't learn to be schizophrenic, you come down with it, like you get diabetes or high blood pressure. Most probably, you inherit it.

If you have a relative with schizophrenia, your chances of contracting it are as follows:

Brother or sister: 8%
Non-identical twin: 12%
One parent: 12%
Both parents: 40%
Identical twin: 48%

The percentages hold true whether you and your relation live in the same house or across the world. These numbers, generated relatively recently, went a long way toward debunking the theory that bad parenting, poverty, social ills or any other "psychological" explanation caused the disease. It is not, as social anthropologist Gregory Bateson proposed in 1960, the result of an "inescapable double bind," mixed messages received from important family members, i.e., hearing assertions of love from your parents while they clench their fists in a contradictory sign of hatred. Schizophrenia is, contrary to Scottish psychiatrist R.D. Laing's 1960s assertion, a real disease, not merely an "experience" or a rational response to an irrational world. And, most definitely, in distinction to Hungarian born and U.S. educated psychiatrist, Thomas Szacz, schizophrenia isn't a "myth." Scasz wrote that, "Mental illness is a myth, whose function is to disguise and thus render more palatable the bitter pill of moral conflicts in human relations."

There are different types of schizophrenia, some worse than others, just like some cancers are worse than others. The disease seems to fall into two basic groups. The first primarily hear voices, think paranoid but organized thoughts and retain most of their basic, albeit aloof, odd or distant personality. When you study their brain structure, not much is grossly wrong. This type of schizophrenia is probably due to a chemical problem inside the brain cells themselves. These people do well on anti-psychotic medications but rarely can be talked into taking them.

They can, with adequate support in times of crisis, lead a fairly normal life: marriage, children and a job for the least afflicted; board-and-care homes and isolation for the more severely diseased. These individuals don't belong in institutions. They rarely wander the streets.

The second group, however, is a different story. These people have the hard-core symptoms of schizophrenia. As if someone hit their brains with a sledge hammer, they choose to wear four layers of ragged, stinking clothes in the summer. They stare vacantly while babbling and defecating in their pants. Freezing to death in public parks and roaming aimlessly down busy highways, they also fill our alleys and steam grates, lost without their persona or intellect. Their problems are serious.

If modern medical scanning techniques are used to examine this second type of schizophrenic brain, significant damage is revealed.

Intelligence tests administered to these people reveal large drops in IQ scores. As well, many of these schizophrenics suffer from "temporal disorientation"; they can't accurately recall the day, month or year, and some misguess their own age by more than five years. As Timothy Crowe, an eminent British psychiatric researcher, has said, "The pattern of intellectual deficits in these patients is difficult to distinguish from that seen in Alzheimer's disease." The original name for schizophrenia, "Dementia Praecox" or early dementia, coined in the nineteenth century, reflects this disease characteristic.

On Computerized Axial Tomography (CAT) scans, schizophrenic brains show ventricular enlargement, the ventricles being hollow spaces through which cerebrospinal fluid flows. The ventricles are expanded because the surrounding tissue has shrunk. This brain loss is more profound in the temporal lobes, the area where hearing and language are processed.

Also, when studied by Positron Emission Tomagraphy (PET) scans, a technique that measures the metabolic capacity of different brain areas, these schizophrenics have decreased function in the "pre-frontal" cortex, the part of the brain that lies just behind the forehead. The pre-frontal cortex handles more complicated "executive" cerebral tasks. These include sophisticated judgment and thinking decisions, exactly what people need to navigate the world of complex human relationships and the problems of daily life. As well, as was first noted by Dr. Elmer Southard of the Boston Psychopathic Hospital in 1915, this second type of schizophrenic brain tends to be perfectly symmetrical, each half being exactly the same size as the other. This isn't normal. Usually one side of the brain, the area that contains your language processing center, is noticeably larger than the other. The language center, where we coordinate input from the outside world and form coherent thinking and speech patterns, doesn't work right in these schizophrenics. This may explain their problems with garbled speech and disorganized thinking. Such abnormalities may be due to brain degeneration or a failure of the organ to develop completely in the first place. Either way, the results are the same: psychosis and dementia—near total brain failure.

As you might imagine, schizophrenics who show the most profound brain cell loss tend to be the most chronic, persistently disabled and psychotic individuals of the group. Not unlike John Doe and a million other Americans like him.

III

For the next two days I put John Doe's writ hearing out of my mind and got down to business as usual. I had ER duty as I did twice weekly, on Tuesdays and Thursdays.

"Hi-Ho, Steverino," Bull said as I walked into the psych ER the following morning. We were the only two people among the day crew old enough to understand the old *Steve Allen Show* reference. Bull was tough, but he had his lighter side.

Yang was right behind me. He grinned at Bull then touched Ten-Trees on the shoulder. "Let's play Cowboys and Indians sometime," he lilted, before disappearing back into the doctors lounge for sign-out rounds.

Ten-Trees tried to remain stoic as ever, but even he couldn't stifle a small smile. "That man is strange," he said finally.

"I think he's sweet on you," Bull added, giving Ten-Trees a gentle chuck under the chin. We were always trying to get Ten-Trees to laugh out loud. It was like acting silly in front of the Buckingham Palace guards.

"I can see it," I said to Bull. "Very handsome couple."

But Ten-Trees wouldn't budge. "This job is strange," he concluded, turning back to some paperwork on the counter in front of him.

Soon everyone was ready for the night crew to sign out. Hundley and Redmond looked haggard as they passed off the eleven remaining patients to Dupree, Yang and Tina. It was the usual stuff: PCP intoxication, amphetamines, cocaine, people found staggering in traffic, threats of suicide, voices, starvation.

"You'd better do this one yourself," Bear said to me as the housestaff finished their presentations.

I raised my eyebrows.

"Kid," Bear said. "Jamal Johnson. He's eight."

"See him with me?" I asked Dupree.

"Certainly," she replied.

Dupree was about to discover that mental illness isn't limited to adults. Children suffer as well.

After the night shift was gone, we set out for the waiting room to collect young Jamal.

IV

With Dupree in tow, I stuck my head out through the psych ER door and into the waiting room.

"Jamal Johnson?" I called, and up from a Bible that lay open in her lap turned the face of an elderly black woman. She smiled and stood as I approached. "I'm Naomi Johnson," she said taking my hand gently. "Jamal is my grandson."

I introduced myself and Dupree, then we headed back to the ER, toward a small interview room where for the next hour we all talked. Jamal was bright and inquisitive. He wore battered but recognizable Air Jordan gym shoes, weathered jeans and a gold Lakers T-shirt. While his clothes weren't new, they were obviously clean and well cared for. As was Jamal. Unfortunately, he was also hyperactive. He had trouble sitting still, twice jumping up to answer the desk phone when it rang. He interrupted my questions. His grandmother had to repeatedly press him back into his chair.

Jamal's tale was the standard kid's story at the Mill. His mother, a cocaine addict, had used drugs throughout her pregnancy, even smoking crack on the way to the hospital in the last stages of labor. "She was a bad seed," Naomi said quietly, barely able to conceal the anger in her voice. "Thank God she's gone now."

"Did she die?" I asked, glancing at Jamal to gauge the pain of his reaction.

"I hope so," Naomi said honestly. Jamal didn't flinch.

"Where is she?" Dupree interjected.

"Out there," Naomi replied, pointing at nowhere in particular.

The County's Department of Children's Services had removed Jamal from the care of his mother who, an anonymous tip alleged, was neglecting him. When the County visited the home, Jamal, age three, was alone and seemed to have been that way for sometime. Urine and feces were everywhere. The refrigerator was empty save a half-melted box of popsicles in the freezer.

Jamal was placed in foster care. By the age of five, he'd been hospitalized twice for broken bones and knocked unconscious three times. He'd been the ward of four different couples before Naomi was even notified. She took immediate action to obtain custody.

Naomi gave us the details of her grandson's tumultuous young life. She had them "in her files" as she put it, patting her purse. She'd become acquainted with the facts pertaining to Jamal's case when she had to fight her daughter for another change of guardianship. Two years previously, the woman had suddenly reappeared, armed with an attorney and a mother's guilt. Before the proceedings could pass beyond the initial evaluation stage, however, she'd disappeared again.

Now, unfortunately, Jamal was facing an even bigger crisis. After the hour had passed, I asked him if Naomi and I could speak alone for a while. He agreed, and Dupree walked the boy out, sitting with him in the lobby.

"How long have you had a bad heart?" I asked Naomi. Her breath was obviously short. I could count the heartbeats pulsing in her neck veins.

She paused and for an instant the serene facade cracked. The despair of a battle about to be lost flashed across her graceful face. "I've had a touch of trouble lately. But I'll be okay. I have to be. Jamal's all this family has left. He's the only hope. Our daughter turned out no good. It's drugs, Doctor," she added, a smoldering anger behind her now fixed eyes. "They ruined everything. You wouldn't understand, but our community wasn't always like this. There was life here once. Energy." Naomi's voice trailed off. We sat in silence for a moment.

"My Walter and I had such plans," she began again with an ironic, almost self-conscious, laugh. Her breath was coming even harder now. "He worked thirty years as a mailman. Dropped dead walking his route not a mile from here." A small tear filled the corner of one eye but was quickly blinked away.

"Our home's paid off. Of course, that don't mean much now. Couldn't sell it if I wanted to. They shoot heroin next door in the front yard. Two men were murdered on the block this month alone."

"We hoped our daughter would to go to college," Naomi continued, her voice barely above a whisper, her breathing more rapid than ever. I was beginning to get worried. She pulled a pill from a small container in her purse and slipped it under her tongue. In a few seconds she seemed refreshed.

"That money all went up the crack pipe, too," Naomi said and sat back. "My husband was a good man. We did our best. It's just me now. And that boy can be a handful."

V

I felt sorry for Naomi and Jamal. There were many similar stories at the Mill, and I knew, if something wasn't done, where things were headed.

The disease affecting Jamal has been known for many years and called different things. Originally named "Minimal Brain Damage" or MBD, it has variously been attributed to food allergies, dietary sugar or poor upbringing. But, as with most mental disorders, the organic, structural nature of hyperactivity is now becoming evident.

The human brain is a delicate organ with intricate and complex wiring, not unlike a computer. If its circuitry is disrupted or incorrectly connected, problems result. The majority of this cerebral network is laid down during pregnancy and early childhood. These are critical periods.

When a pregnant woman contracts certain diseases, like German measles or syphilis, or when bad chromosomes are passed on to an unborn child, as with Down's syndrome, the unfortunate infant will have external problems that are readily apparent to everyone. There are gross structural aberrations in the youngster's brain. The trouble is in the "hardware."

Intrauterine exposure to drugs, alcohol, narcotics and, specifically, cocaine, also results in hardware damage, but the changes are more subtle. The machine looks normal but just doesn't work correctly.

When early childhood neglect combines with pre-natal substance exposure, the effects are double. The human brain isn't complete when you're born. Some of the more complicated and subtle intellectual functions are only acquired as a person grows. Neglect and maltreatment warp these final touches to a child's "programming." It adds a software "glitch" into the mix. Instead of developing reasoning, empathy, judgment, insight and behavior control, a child suffers from inattention, hyperactivity and impulsivity. These characteristics are grouped together into what's known as "Attention Deficit Hyperactivity Disorder" or "ADHD." A subgroup of kids with ADHD gets depressed. This combination of emotional distress and distractibility make staying out of trouble difficult. A fair proportion of ADHD children becomes juvenile delinquents and ends up in prison.

It's a complicated problem. Not all hyperactive kids were tainted with drugs or ignored. It just seems to happen sometimes, just as a number of neglected and abused youngsters don't get ADHD. But in our neighborhood, around the Mill, the percentage of children with ADHD is high, as is the incidence of substance abuse and parental dereliction.

For kids with ADHD, receiving early treatment is paramount. The only chance for many of them is medication, specifically drugs called "psychostimulants." These are medicines that act like amphetamines. Ritalin is the best known. Cylert is another. For unknown reasons, they calm hyperactive kids. A child can then sit still in class and get an education, one of the only tickets out of the ghetto.

As with all decisions regarding medications and children, however, there are many things to consider before prescribing them. All drugs have side effects, which must be weighed against potential benefits. Some children on stimulants develop tics, abnormal and repetitive muscle twitching. Many have difficulty sleeping. Of a more serious nature, there's a controversy about chronic stimulant use stunting a child's growth.

Before deciding on the use of medicine for Jamal, I needed additional data, but before even that, I had to ask Naomi the question
that had been obvious since we'd first sat down.

"What will happen to Jamal if you become too ill to care for
him?" I said straight out.

Now Naomi's eyes took on a desperate, pleading quality. "The
boy isn't right. That's why we're here. You've got to help him."

"There are medications to treat..." I began, attempting to ease
the woman's pain.

"The issue isn't medicine," Naomi interjected firmly. "We're
talking about when I die. You've got to see that Jamal doesn't go back
to his mother. He needs to be placed in a decent home. If not, he'll
end up like all the rest of them, dead or in jail. The court will listen to a
doctor." For the first time, a tear came to Naomi's eye that couldn't
be blinked away.

A lot of things were going through my mind. I was thinking
about Naomi and her dreams which, seemingly, lay in ruins. Then
there was Jamal. The kid had started life ten yards behind the pack
and was in danger of dropping from the race altogether. My mind
turned to my own boys—Jake and Mike—and the plans Linda and I
had for their futures. Then finally I remembered a lesson someone
had taught me when I was a resident-in-training. It went something
like this: You may not be able to solve all the troubles of the ghetto,
but you can, occasionally, fix one problem for one person.

"I promise Jamal will be taken care of," I blurted.

This sort of thing has plagued me most of my life. It's probably
one of the reasons I became a physician in the first place. Jamal and
Naomi's situation wasn't right, and I felt compelled to repair it. I
couldn't save all the ghetto kids from going down the drain, but
maybe one could be snatched away—the one whose grandmother was
sitting in that small ER conference room nobly struggling for breath
and her family's dignity. In a strange way, I felt I owed it to her.

Naomi visibly relaxed. "Thank you," she said.

Am I Insane?

"YOU DID WHAT!?" Bear said, a cheeseburger poised in front of his mouth.

I always consulted Bear on my tougher cases and thought I would ask him about Jamal.

"You did what!?" he said again when I didn't answer immediately. People from other booths were beginning to turn and look.

"I promised the boy's grandmother I'd look after him when she died," I whispered. "You know, see that he gets placed somewhere decent."

We were at a local McDonald's, one of the few businesses open in the area. "You did what?" Bear said a third time. His burger hadn't moved.

"You heard me."

"Are you insane?" Bear's sunglasses were aimed directly at me. I could see my reflection in the lenses.

"Right now, I'm not so sure."

"Jesus, Steve," Bear huffed, setting down the sandwich and wiping his mouth with one rapid sweep of a napkin. "You've been working for the County long enough. When is the little light going to go on? Won't you guys ever learn? Christ almighty!" He threw his napkin to the floor.

I'd never seen Bear like this. I thought he was going to hit me. Yet, I wasn't as stupid as it sometimes appeared. A nerve had been struck that ran deeper than Jamal Johnson.

"'You guys?'" I asked.

Bear took a deep breath, grabbing the edge of the small Formica table. "Sorry," he said, exhaling. "I didn't mean anything. But you should realize that life for ghetto kids is just one letdown after another. Lots of people promise you everything all the time, then at the last minute, it gets pulled away."

"There's no knight in shining armor going to ride in and solve your problems for you." Bear's voice was rising; people were staring again. "Jamal understands more about living here than you ever will. He's going to end up in some crap situation no matter what you do. What happens if the court doesn't give him back to his mother which, incidentally, they probably will? Are you going to take in a hyperactive black kid? Your wife would love that. 'By the way dear, I couldn't help but notice that you've brought a young boy home from the office.'" Bear's voice changed into his best dullard's drawl. "'Well, Sweetheart, I made a little promise one day at work...'" He shook his head.

"But his mother abused him. The court will never give him back to her."

"They can and most likely will," Bear said, seeming to have regained control. "Hundreds of cases go through the juvenile system every year exactly like this. They'll be thrilled if a relative shows up at all. What do you think their placement options are? Do you imagine there's some huge, untapped reservoir of stable families willing to take in a disturbed child? I mean, look around." Bear waved toward a nearby window.

At that moment, a drunken man across the street stumbled and lurched face down into the gutter. After wiping the blood from his nose, he fought back up onto the curb and continued on his way, crawling down the sidewalk.

"The juvenile court doesn't give a shit about the people down here," Bear continued angrily. "The mental health court doesn't give a shit about our patients. The County, State and Feds don't care either. No one gives a crap about Jamal, you, me, the neighborhood or the hospital. The whole place could burn tomorrow, and all you'd hear is a collective sigh of relief."

I didn't know what to say.

"It takes an act of God to get out of this pesthole," Bear concluded disgustedly.

After a moment I said, "You got out, Bear. Was that Divine intervention?"

"That's nobody's business but mine," he replied.

II

I hadn't lived in LA for long, but I imagined that what Bear said about the ghetto was true. But LA isn't just the ghetto. Where my family lived, although physically proximate, was very different. In reality, there is no defining location or statement about LA, it's such a diverse and incongruous place.

We live in the city of Torrance in an area called the South Bay near Redondo and Manhattan Beach, just north of the heavy industrial ports of San Pedro and Long Beach. Torrance is a working class city full of many long-time residents mixed with a huge population of recent immigrants.

Ours is a two story condominium complex. Across the way lives a Japanese sushi chef, his wife and two children, below them a couple from Laos. To the left is a Sikh family recently emigrated from India and next over, a group of Chinese fundamentalist Christians. Every so often, at night, their apartment fills with other Chinese Christians (you can gauge the size of the gathering by the number of shoes piled outside the door), and they sing. Loudly, in Chinese, while lying prostrate on the living room floor. I walked over and peeked in the window once.

A retired pair resides next door with a grown daughter. Above us are two stockbrokers. And down the way, on the second floor, is a young couple, teachers I suspect, who own a bird.

This, however, is no ordinary bird. It's one of those big South American things. "Birdie," as he's known, stands almost two feet tall, including tail feathers. Birdie also has a strange habit. Beginning every morning and continuing to nightfall, he starts at the top of the second-story stair railing and "surfs" down to the ground floor, then, like a tightrope walker, he walks back up the banister and slides down again, flapping his wings and screaming. More than once I've run outside thinking someone was being strangled. Our complex can be an unusual place.

The spring of 1992 was unusual for LA in general. It was the time of the Rodney King trial. The previous summer, all the world had seen the videotape of King, a black man, getting clubbed by a ring of angry white LAPD officers after a long, high-speed car chase. The cops, charged with brutality, were now being prosecuted.

Owing to the intensity of local sentiment, the proceedings had been moved from LA to Simi Valley, an all-white suburb north of the city. Everyone was tense, as if fifteen million people were waiting for the other shoe to drop. The officers were guilty, that was certain. What effect their conviction would have on police morale was unknown. That the jury could go the other way wasn't even a consideration.

None of this bothered me as I arrived home that night. My mind was elsewhere. I was still upset about Jamal, about Bear, about a lot of things.

I was quiet at dinner and afterwards, attempting to sort things out, went for a walk. It didn't help.

Later that night, with the boys in bed, I felt the need for some support, some reassurance that maybe Bear had overreacted and, perhaps, my decision about Jamal hadn't been so bad after all.

Linda was sitting in front of the TV when I turned down the volume and ran the basics of my conversation with Naomi Johnson by her. She listened attentively, then reaching for the remote control and looking me straight in the eyes, she said, "Are you insane?" I can't remember her ever sounding more serious.

It was a low point. I swore things could only improve.

III

Jamal Johnson wasn't mentioned again all weekend. Linda gratefully called a momentary truce in our smoldering skirmish over living in LA and my working at the Mill, so things went smoothly. On Saturday we walked the boys to the park; I hit them fly balls, and we feasted on pizza. That Sunday, Linda and I took in a movie and talked on the phone for an hour to our daughter.

On Monday morning, owing to the fact that my job can sometimes be messy, I didn't wear a tie to work. In fact, I'd become rather infamous around the hospital for a casual style of dress, usually a golf shirt with Levi's or slacks. I had one favorite shirt. It was a nice, well-washed, off red. The shirt had a pocket on the left breast to which my hospital ID badge clipped. About every six months, however, I would put it on and wonder where the pocket had gone. As Linda politely puts it, I'm frequently "not in tune with my environment." During the day, I'd keep trying to put a pen in my pocket and wonder again where it had gone. Or, I finally would conclude, I probably had two red shirts, one with a pocket and one without. The dilemma would invariably be cleared up by lunchtime when one of the housestaff or a colleague would tug at the exposed tag on the neck of my shirt and inform me that I had it on inside out. Glancing down inside my collar I would find the missing pocket.

Similarly, every morning, I would locate my belt before deciding which other clothes to wear. One day it was my black belt, hence a dark outfit, another A.M. it would be my brown belt—a light outfit. It was an entire year before Linda pointed out that, in fact, I only owned one belt and that it was reversible.

In short, life's small details, car keys, wallets, ID tags and glasses, are the bane of my existence. It's the rare morning in which ten minutes isn't spent looking for something. But that Monday, miraculously, everything was found in short order. As I pulled into the parking lot at work I was feeling pretty good, until I spotted Tina, standing at the curb.

"Ready?" I said, as she opened the front passenger door.

"I guess," Tina replied, warily inspecting my car. "Do you need shots to ride in this thing?"

I've never been much of an auto buff. To me they just get you where you want to go and, with two athletic sons, I was constantly hauling a herd of sweaty, dirt-stained kids home from games, to and from Taco Bell, to the batting cage, etc. Making a long story short, my 1987 Toyota was a trash heap.

"Very funny," I said wheeling back into the street, heading toward the freeway. "Just to be safe, are your tetanus boosters up to date?"

We made jokes, but Tina and I were both nervous. We were going to John Doe's writ hearing.

Court 95, LA County's Mental Health Court facility, is a little past downtown, in a small industrial strip across the street from the new Metro Link railyard in a part of town called Chavez Ravine, which sports fans will recognize as the site of Dodger Stadium. The ballpark is on the other side of the train tracks and up a hill. Tina and I could see the right field light standards as we parked.

The court building itself is low and unimposing, actually a converted pickle factory. There's no marker or sign outside. You have to know it is there. The sight of twenty ragged, mumbling people waiting in an outside courtyard trying to bum cigarettes from every person passing by does act as a tip-off.

The utilitarian exterior of the courthouse matches an equally prosaic interior. A large waiting room is filled with more tattered people, an occasional family member and a cadre of attorneys who regularly flit in and out. Sections of the daily paper and old magazines lie scattered along rows of benches. The courtroom itself is also standard issue, definitely more *Cagney and Lacey* than *LA Law*.

At 8:45 A.M., Tina and I registered at the district attorney's office and met briefly with Rick Barnes, the man who would argue our case before the judge. He gave Tina a smile. They were about the same age.

I'd known Barnes since I had first come to court as a resident. He'd handled lots of my *habeas corpus* writs before. As was the case with all the attorneys in the DA's office, Barnes was genuinely concerned about the patients we brought him. With vigor and compassion, he represented the hospital's request for continued treatment.

Barnes reviewed our situation, asked us a few questions and wrote down the answers. "We'll see," he said. "You know how Judge Cohen can be." Then he strode away. We walked back into the lobby to wait for John Doe's case to be called.

It was 9:00 when Tina and I sat in the busy waiting room. She found the front section of the *LA Times* and began reading. I fished a copy of *Modern Maturity* off the floor.

By 11:00, I'd read every article in the magazine. Tina was finished with the newspaper and had paced around the room innumerable times. She was now sitting beside me, hands cupped beneath her chin. The superior court operated on its own schedule. Once, I'd waited until 4:30 P.M. for a hearing to begin.

After a while, I saw Barnes standing near the courtroom door and walked over.

"Mr. Doe here yet?" he asked, checking his watch.

"No," I answered, looking back toward the main door. The van that brought patients from ours and other County hospitals to court was often late.

Barnes glanced quickly at some papers. "This Doe guy's a real mess?"

"When the cops brought him in covered with excrement; he didn't look human."

Barnes shook his head. "Poor man."

I scanned the waiting room. It was filled with other patients like John Doe, some from private hospitals, many from the local jails. They all had the same bedraggled look about them. "Why do you do this?" I asked. "Couldn't you have a big office on Wilshire?"

Half smiling, Barnes nodded. "Probably. But I like to think we're doing something important. Something that makes a difference, helping these people get better."

I was curious from where Barnes' interest stemmed. "You get formal training in mental health issues in law school?"

"No," he replied. "You pick up most things on your own."

"Is it personal? Someone sick in your family? A friend?"

"My brother," Barnes said without hesitation. "He's schizo-phrenic. Took off four years ago. No one's heard from him since. Damn near killed my parents..." He fell silent.

Standing next to Barnes, I looked at the mass of neglected humanity in the lobby and thought that somewhere outside another courtroom or walking down a distant freeway was Rick Barnes' brother.

"What do you think causes mental illness?" I asked.

Barnes thought for a second, "I'm not sure. Maybe it's a chemical thing. Who knows?"

His answer made me sad. Even those intimately involved with deciding the fates of these sick people didn't really understand their disease.

"What do you think about our country's mental health system?" I asked finally.

"It sucks," he said, then checked the time again and, touching me on the shoulder, walked away.

At 11:15, the County van finally arrived with John Doe and eight other patients. Watching him walk through the door, I knew we were doomed. His hair was cut. He was clean-shaven and had on fresh hospital clothes. When he saw Tina, he waved.

To be sure, the man was crazy as ever. We spoke briefly before going into the courtroom proper. "I know you're in this with the FBI," John Doe hissed, peering around conspiratorially. Certain that no one else could hear he went on, "When this Nazi cunt judge releases me, I'm going to get even with you and that Jacobs bitch. Count on it." With that he turned and walked through the courtroom doors. The blood drained from my face.

"What'd he say?" Tina said, walking up.

"Nothing." We followed John Doe inside.

I was extremely unsettled. While threats from patients weren't that frequent, I always took them seriously. My family didn't live far from the hospital, certainly within walking distance, especially for a man on a mission. As the bailiff stood to announce the end of a short recess, I felt something cold on my neck. Reaching up, I wiped away a small drop of sweat.

"All rise," proclaimed the bailiff, and from an unmarked door to the side of an imposing judicial bench, in walked Judge Marvin Cohen, a short, kind-faced man. Dressed in a black robe, he smiled at the bailiff, then to the assembled attorneys and took his seat.

"In the matter of John Doe," Cohen began, and our patient, obviously having done this numerous times before, rose from his front row seat in the gallery, passed through a small swinging gate held open by the bailiff and took his place next to the public defender at one of two long tables in front of the judge. Barnes sat at the other table.

Barnes spoke first. "I call Dr. Seager," he said. Taking a breath, I looked at Tina then went through the same hinged door and stood to Cohen's right beside the witness stand.

"Raise your right hand," the bailiff said. "Do you solemnly swear that the testimony you are about to give before this court is the truth, the whole truth and nothing but the truth, so help you God?

"Yes," I affirmed and sat down.

"Nice to see you again, Dr. Seager," Cohen said.

"Nice to be here," I replied for lack of anything better to say.

Cohen formalized his tone. "Proceed."

After the preliminaries of spelling my name, stating my position as a ward chief on the psychiatric in-patient unit and verifying that I was board certified in the medical specialty of psychiatry, I recounted how John Doe had been picked up walking down the freeway. I confirmed that he had been feces-and-pest-ridden at the time and that he'd been admitted in similar condition eighty-four times in the past four years.

"What's your diagnosis?" Barnes asked.

"Chronic schizophrenia," I stated.

"Does Mr. Doe remain persistently psychotic?"

"Yes."

"And does that condition, in your opinion, preclude him from providing for his own food, clothing and shelter?"

"The man shits in his pants, wanders on the freeway and eats garbage."

"Would that be a 'yes'?" Barnes asked.

"Yes," I said firmly.

"What are your plans for the continuing care of Mr. Doe?"

"Clearly he can't look after himself. If he returns to the streets he'll most likely die in the not-too-distant future. He needs a conservatorship and long-term treatment at the state hospital."

"That's all," Barnes said.

"Ms. Perkins," Cohen called, turning to the public defender.

I braced for an icy blast. The public defenders were a hard-nosed bunch.

Ms. Perkins (I didn't know her first name) was a waspish, thin woman, a Carol Burnett look-alike. She twirled a pair of glasses in her hand as she spoke. "Is Mr. Doe eating hospital food?" she asked.

"Yes, but..."

"Thank you."

"Is he dressed in an appropriate manner?" Perkins continued.

"He's wearing hospital clothes. We had to burn what he came in with."

Perkins paused for a second. The glasses stopped spinning. "In your opinion, is hospital clothing appropriate for a person in the hospital?"

"Of course, he's dressed appropriately and eating!" I wanted to shout. "Our nurses dress and feed him." I often thought we should withhold medication, baths and clean clothes from our patients so the courts could see just how bad these people looked when left to their own devices. But, naturally, we couldn't do that.

"Yes," I said finally. "He's dressed appropriately."

"Where does Mr. Doe live?" Perkins went on.

"He claims to live in an abandoned building on 39th and Crenshaw. But..."

"Thank you, Dr. Seager," Perkins said curtly. "That's all, your Honor."

"You're excused," Cohen intoned, dismissing me.

I left the witness chair and retook my seat next to Tina. "We're goners," I whispered, sitting down.

Following me, John Doe took the stand. He gave an address for the condemned building and stated the location of two restaurant dumpsters from which he claimed to eat regularly. He said he'd take his medication and keep his clothes clean. He didn't slap anybody. Inside of twenty minutes the whole affair was over. John Doe was released.

A few things struck me while watching John Doe testify. The first was Judge Cohen. He was unfailingly polite, even deferential to my sick patient. He listened attentively and always addressed the man as "Mister Doe" or "Sir." He seemed to care about John Doe in a personal way, which made his decision to grant the writ all the more confusing. I needed to talk with Cohen at some point.

The other thing that got my attention was Ms. Perkins. The public defenders had always been just adversaries to be overcome, but now I began wondering about her and the other attorneys like her. Why, I thought, does she do what she does? What was her slant on this whole court/homeless/mentally ill business? There had to be a reason for her rigorous advocacy. Did she see the larger picture or ever view things from our end of the spectrum? Did she understand what it's like to hose lice and feces off another human being?

The last thing that hit me was more personal. John Doe was now a free man. Suddenly, there was a knot in my stomach the size of a basketball.

"Congratulations, Mr. Doe," Perkins said after Cohen's ruling. She wore the smile of a job well done. John Doe turned to go.

"See you later," he sneered, strolling confidently past me and out of the courtroom.

John Doe was right—we would see each other again. Neither of us, however, could have imagined how soon that would actually be.

Death by Spa

TINA AND I WERE STANDING OUTSIDE COURT 95. Ours had been one of the last morning cases called. Nearly everyone was gone, and we were alone on the sidewalk.

"What now?" she said quietly.

"Now nothing. Back to work."

We walked a few steps in silence. "Did I do anything wrong?" Tina asked, not looking up.

We both stopped. "You did a wonderful job," I said sincerely. "John Doe got the best care possible."

"I tried so hard," she whispered. "Everything seems so pointless." She looked crushed.

"It's just a ridiculous system," I said as we began walking again.

"What will happen to John Doe?"

The answer to that one was tough. "He'll wander in traffic, get another infection or murdered, maybe freeze to death. Something."

We got to the car, I unlocked the door and Tina slid inside. Just then, the County van rolled by, the one taking John Doe back to the hospital where, after signing a few papers, he would leave. As it passed, I glanced in through the rear window. John Doe was staring back. He gave me the finger. "Nazi cunt," he mouthed silently.

When Tina and I arrived at the hospital, John Doe was gone. Inside of an hour, a new patient had been sent up from the Psych ER whom I assigned to Tina. Getting right back into the fray is always the best cure for disappointment.

Mr. Tran, a Vietnamese man of forty-five, arrived on the ward in a wheelchair with a large ice bag on his lap. I called and spoke to Bull.

He said the man had come in with an elaborate twine harness attached to his penis, pulled so tightly that he'd nearly cut off the organ's blood supply.

As odd as this story sounds, it's not that rare among Southeast Asian populations. Mr. Tran suffered from *Koro*, a delusional belief that one's genitals are contracting into the body. The delusions aren't so bad, but the contraptions the victims construct to fight them are.

Koro is one of an interesting group of psychiatric disorders called "Culture-Bound" syndromes, which means they tend to be specific to a single group of people. Eskimos experience *Piblokto* or "Arctic Hysteria," a condition in which someone, usually a woman, becomes briefly but acutely psychotic, screaming, tearing off her clothing and running out into the tundra. *Wihtigo*, a disorder among the American Plains Indians, is the belief that any abdominal discomfort indicates the individual is being transformed into a flesh-eating monster, a *wihtigo*.

The most famous syndrome of this group is *Amok*. During an *Amok* attack, someone, generally of Malaysian origin, experiences a bout of intense rage. The victim runs wildly through the streets, stabbing anyone who crosses his path. The police in the area carry "*Amok* sticks," a long pole forked at one end, allowing them to subdue the insane person by pinning him around the neck against a wall. *Amok* is also short-lived. Unfortunately, upon recovering, the patients often commit suicide when confronted with the havoc they've wrecked. A good example of *Amok* can be seen in the Woody Allen movie *Radio Days* in which a neighbor, accurately portrayed with a knife, runs screaming down the street. We've adopted the word into our own vernacular. When someone acts in a strange or violent way, we say he has "run amok."

Tina looked down the hall toward Mr. Tran who'd dumped his ice bag on the ground and was pulling wildly at the crotch of his pants.

"Here we go again," she said as we ran toward him.

II

That afternoon I left a little later than usual. Walking through the nearly empty parking lot toward my car, I felt a sudden shudder, unable to get John Doe out of my mind.

It was strangely quiet around our condo complex when I got home. Birdie wasn't out. There were no children on the walk, and everyone had finished eating; there wasn't a single barbecue burning.

Approaching our front door, I dropped my keys at the sound of footsteps behind me. I gasped and spun around. My elderly neighbor gasped too. She put a hand over her chest.

"I'm so sorry," I said, fumbling for my key ring then stepping over to be certain the woman was all right.

"I'm fine," she said with a breathy smile. "You just startled me." Then she patted me on the cheek. "Linda's right. You've gotta get another job."

For obvious reasons, of late I hadn't been discussing much about work with my wife, and I certainly had no intention of mentioning the threat from John Doe. I was so obviously distracted during dinner, though, she asked me twice what was wrong.

"I must be coming down with something," I lied, picking at my food.

Around ten, after the boys had been put to bed and while Linda watched a cable channel movie, I changed into a pair of shorts and grabbed a towel from the hall closet.

"I'm going to soak in the spa," I said, and Linda nodded.

One of the nice things about southern California is the beautiful night weather. Often, when life's stresses start to overwhelm me, I'll fire up the hot tub we share with our neighbors, let the warm water flow over me, lean back and stare at the stars.

The sky was moonless and dark as I swung open the gate and entered the spa enclave. Flipping a switch on the nearby wall, an underwater light clicked on in the small round pool, and air jets began to furiously churn the hot, steamy water. Anticipating the comforting warmth, I finally forgot all about John Doe.

As I stepped into the water, I sensed something wasn't right. The ground beneath my feet began to move. Suddenly, I lost my footing completely, as if rolling off a log. Falling hard, I cracked my forehead against the side of the spa. Blood trickled into my eyes, and I went blank.

When I awoke—after how long?—my neck was cradling the lip of the spa. I struggled to clear my head.

Roiling and frothing over my body, the water had turned a deep burgundy. All that blood couldn't be mine. Reeling backwards, like someone recoiling from a poised snake, I pulled away and stood on the concrete deck.

There, at the bottom of the spa, eyes open, glaring exactly as he'd done earlier that morning, lay John Doe. I'd stepped on him.

I didn't panic or scream. In the medical ER, death had been too constant a companion for it to evoke such a reaction. The man's skin color was slate blue. There would be no need for CPR or any rescue attempt. He was long since dead. The cops would have to fish him out.

Before summoning help, however, I stared for a moment at John Doe. The bizarre coincidence and tragedy of the moment struck me. By what widely divergent paths had both of us come to be in the same spa, that exact night? Each with cuts on our heads. One alive. One dead.

John Doe had eaten garbage, existed on the cruel streets and suffered atrocious indignities. In contrast, I'd lived like a king. Accounting for this enormous disparity, there was but one distinction between us; he'd gotten sick, and I hadn't.

Standing and staring, as morbid and frightening as it was, I couldn't help but wonder, "How had he found my house? What if he hadn't hit his head? Why hadn't I drowned?" In that instant, I forged a connection with John Doe. I had to find out more about him.

By then Linda was at the spa gate. "Are you all right?" She was peering in through the metal rails. "You've been gone..."

She let out a sharp scream and covered her mouth.

"Don't come in," I said walking toward her. "Call the police."

After what seemed forever, three officers arrived followed closely by an ambulance. As Linda pressed a towel to my bloody forehead, John Doe's body was dragged from the water and placed on a gurney. His face covered with a sheet, he was wheeled away. The attendants slid the corpse into the back of the ambulance, closed the doors and, without flashing lights, drove off.

As a small clutch of people gathered around the spa entrance, Linda and I gave the police our statements. Unfortunately, there wasn't much to tell. Although John Doe had been my patient for nearly two weeks, I didn't know any more about him then than when he'd first come through the psych ER doors.

III

The next morning our local paper mentioned the drowning of John Doe. A picture taken outside the condo complex accompanied the story. In all the hubbub we hadn't noticed a photographer.

At work, I felt strangely reticent about discussing the incident. Explaining the Band-Aid on my forehead as the result of a fall, I let it go at that. Tina and I would have to talk over John Doe's death, but it wasn't going to be then. My thoughts and emotions were too jumbled. So, the day proceeded as usual. I saw patients and talked about cases with the housestaff; my conversation with the nurses was amicable and light. I didn't notice the knot in my stomach until the drive home.

When I entered our condo, Linda was standing out on the small verandah just off of the living room. A half-empty wine bottle stood beside her on a wire-legged table. She didn't turn as the glass door slid open. This was a bad sign.

From the patio, if you look carefully between the other units and just over the roof of a nearby restaurant, you can see the lights of the distant city. I'd spent my share of time, over the past few years, watching the night, listening to the lives of other people go by.

Silently reclosing the door I went in to say hello to the boys. Ages eleven and eight, they were in their bedroom hunched over two omnipresent Nintendo controls as a steady stream of explosions and electronic music emanated from a nearby television screen.

"Is your mom okay?" I asked when they finally looked up.

"I guess," Mike, the older boy, said, ripping off a burst of machine gun fire. "She showed us the picture from the paper."

"You really knew that guy?" Jake, the youngest, asked.

"Yes, Jake," I answered. "He was a patient of mine."

"Pretty weird," he said, turning again to the game.

Mike looked at Jake then at me. He didn't say anything.

"Can we still use the spa?" Jake asked.

"Of course."

"As long as there aren't any more dead guys in it," Mike added, his eyes returning to the TV screen.

I left the boys to their computerized mayhem and walked into the living room. Sitting on the couch, I put my head back and tried to sort through the events of the past day. The patio door opened and Linda walked by. "You've got to get out of that place," she said. "We're leaving LA."

There was so much that needed to be said. About how confused I was. About how I'd begun to question the purpose of my job at the Mill. Maybe the idea of public psychiatry was a joke. I wanted to say how stunned and angry I was that the court released John Doe and within hours he was dead. I wanted to ask Linda what this said about the mental health system, about me, about all of us.

I wanted to say a lot of things but never got the chance. "Just get out of there, Steve," Linda reiterated walking down the hall and slamming the door to our bedroom.

Linda's mood settled over the entire house. The boys stayed out of sight. Watching TV didn't help. I walked out onto the patio. The night air was warm and still. Pulling up a deck chair, I sat down; my mind wandered.

Strangely, with all the tension and upheaval surrounding John Doe's death, I became fixated on learning his real name. He'd always just been John Doe, street schizophrenic. As the evening passed and I continued to gaze numbly into the sky, that phrase began to haunt me. "Where the hell did the term 'street schizophrenic' come from anyway?" I wondered. More specifically, when did we start tolerating such a thing? When did we begin allowing mentally crippled people to live like that?

Feeling the knot in my stomach, I walked back inside, made myself a tall drink and laid on the couch. When I opened my eyes, the sun was up.

That morning, Linda and I got the kids off to school, but our conversation was rote. She wouldn't look me in the eye. Her jaw was set. I dressed and drove to work.

During in-patient rounds, Yang, Dupree, Tina, the staff and I sat around the large conference room table for an hour clinically, dispassionately discussing our patients, the next group of John Does who would, despite our best efforts, eventually find their way back to the streets. John Doe wasn't mentioned. The wound was too fresh. We needed a little time.

Afterwards Tina stopped me in the hall. "I saw the article in the paper," she said in a tone of confusion mixed with anger. "Why didn't you tell me?"

"I'm sorry," was the best answer I could muster. "Everything's a little overwhelming right now."

Tina and I stood for what seemed an eternity. Teacher and pupil. Friends. We were both hurting. Thankfully, she broke the silence. "Will there be a funeral? What exactly happens when street people die?"

Despite my having worked in the County mental health system for five years, this was a question for which I had no answer. Our social workers placed most patients in board-and-care homes after discharge from the ward. We occasionally found a family member willing to take in a sick relative. Community shelters were always an option of last resort. After that I really hadn't thought much about what happened to our patients. Many of them eventually wandered back to the streets and certainly some of them died, but like most people, I figured someone else took care of it. Tina's question bothered me.

"I haven't the faintest idea," I had to reply.

At that moment, however, with Tina standing before me, I decided to find out. Bear would have the answer. If anything concerned the ghetto, he knew about it. Late that afternoon, I found him in the psych ER. We sat in the doctors lounge. I began with John Doe's name.

"Names don't matter," Bear said. "It's not a relevant issue. They connect you to society. This means Social Security numbers, income tax forms and all that shit. Society cut the mentally ill loose a long time ago. They're on their own. Why should they be concerned about names?"

"But doesn't a name relate you to your family?"

"Families don't like it, but they eventually give up as well," Bear answered. "They can't care for these people. They try over and over. Remember the elderly Samoan woman who got the hell beat out her with a baseball bat? The chronically mentally ill are too disorganized and unpredictable to have in your house. State hospitals are closed. What's a family supposed to do?"

All these familiar questions without answers were irritating me. I got to the point. "What happens when street schizophrenics die? What will they do with John Doe? Are there funeral services?"

Bear laughed out loud. "Yeah, Steve, they do it up real big. Usually over at Forest Lawn. You can't believe what the County spends on flowers alone. And the limo bills? Forget it." Bear was laughing so hard he had to lift his sunglasses and wipe his eyes. "Sorry, man," he said finally. "It's just that sometimes you..."

That was enough. "Sometimes I what, Bear?" I snapped. "Show a grain of humanity? Sorry I'm not hip enough. Sorry I wasn't raised in the ghetto. That just wasn't an option in Ogden, Utah."

Bear grew more serious. "What I was going to say, is that sometimes you forget about the mentally ill's true place in society; they're beneath the bottom of the barrel. But the way you are is okay. Sometimes I wish I could forget too."

I regretted losing my temper and asked about the funerals again.

This time Bear was direct. "Of course, there won't be a funeral."

"I don't understand. Don't they get buried?"

"Some do."

"And the others?"

"Burned up. Maybe twenty or thirty at a time. LA's a big county. Lots of crazy people die every year. Cremating them individually would cost a fortune."

My stomach tightened up one more notch. "That can't be true," I argued naively. "It sounds like concentration camp stuff. Give me a break."

"This is public knowledge," Bear replied. "A mortician went to prison a few years back for that very thing. Only he got stupid. He burned a few normal people in with the nuts. People whose families actually checked up on things like, 'Are those really Grandpa's ashes in the urn?'"

Startlingly, Bear was right. I'd read the story in the newspaper myself. Back then, however, the anger of the relatives had concerned me, the indignity they must have suffered. Now there was another side to consider. What about those who'd been used as kindling?

"Your concentration camp analogy isn't too far off either," Bear said. "If you think about it."

I didn't want to do that but found myself unable to stop. "You said some people get buried?"

"Yeah, that was in the paper too." Bear said, tilting his head at the faint sound of screeching tires in the distance. "Every so often they dump a bunch of dead lunatics in the ground along with some regular dead guy, bill the family then charge the County, too. Sounds like a money maker to me."

I had a terrible taste in my mouth but said nothing.

"Even with this stuff going on right under our noses," Bear continued. "We choose to ignore it. You've seen those shit-stained guys laying around the parks. What did you think happened when they died? They're invisible. They're nothing. We don't care about them when they're alive, why should we be concerned when they die? We don't pay to feed 'em, why pay to bury 'em?"

"Because they're people, Bear, human beings."

"Wrong," Bear said firmly. "They *were* human beings. Now they're 'transients' or 'street people.' The day they got crazy is the day they died. The rest is just playing out the string. In America today," he continued. "You come down with bad schizophrenia, you're going to starve or freeze and get burned like cordwood."

IV

The rest of the day dissolved in a numb haze of bad feelings. It was as if Bear had been speaking specifically about me. Often driving past brain-diseased people on the road, I'd looked away as they huddled under freeway bridges. While walking, I'd crossed the street to avoid even the chance of speaking with one outside the safe confines of the hospital—in the "wild," as it were. I'd done all the things most people do, ignoring the mentally ill like everybody else.

But I was much more to blame than the average person. After all, the County paid me to care for them. During my years at County General and now the Mill, I'd seen a thousand homeless mentally ill patients, medicated them, cleaned them up, then sent them out the door again. Now the situation was starting to upset me. "What's happening here?" I thought. The answer continued to elude me.

On the way home, as the sunset sky was turning California-seaside purple, I stopped at a traffic light and happened to glance into a vacant lot across the street. On the car radio Gogi Grant was singing "The Tennessee Waltz." In the center of the nearby rubble, a filthy, shirtless man twirled, arms to the heavens, in unintended unison with the music.

Even after the light changed, I couldn't take my eyes off the man. As the music stopped, the DJ's voiced jarred me back into reality.

"I'm sorry," I said, pulling away while the dancer continued his private steps under the darkening sky.

 **Kung Fu Fighting**

THE TENSION WAS PALPABLE as I arrived home that night. My wife was on an entirely different wavelength now.

"You said this Mill job would only be temporary," Linda stated as I walked in the front door. Her tone had a rehearsed quality to it.

"I know..."

"You said you'd start looking for something else right away. And have you?" she demanded.

"Not..."

"No, you haven't." She cut me off, her voice even and firm. "Well, that's it, Steve. We can't go on like this. I can't live with gangs anymore, in a place where you're terrified to walk at night. Where cops beat black men senseless. Where people eat out of garbage cans. And my sons will not grow up in a town where sick men drown in your spa."

I reached out to put an arm around Linda but she stiffly spun away. "You'd better understand how serious this is," she said, her resolve apparent. "We have to get out of here. You can't work in that human sewer anymore..." Finally the tears came.

I felt horrible. Linda had been raised in rural Idaho and had no intention of making LA her permanent home. Despite knowing this, I'd gone blithely about my personal career agenda even when it wasn't clear what that agenda was. Our lives—mine, Linda's and the children's—had always gone my way. They'd taken all the turns I'd decided to take. Gone down my roads. It was a sobering experience watching Linda as she wept.

"I'll start looking for something tomorrow," I said. "We'll get out of the city. I promise."

II

There were two calls on my list of things to do before starting the next day's ward shift. The number of a physician placement service was second. First was tracking down John Doe's name. The need to notify his family suddenly had become paramount.

"I'm calling about the homeless man who drowned last Tuesday," I said, beginning with the county morgue, figuring a quick connection to the right people would get me what I wanted. "He was listed as John Doe."

"Yeah, so?" a disinterested woman replied from the other end.

"I'd like to find his real name."

"You family?"

"Yes," I lied in the interest of expedience.

"Then you should know his name," the woman said and began to hang up.

"Wait! Wait!" I pleaded, hoping the woman was still listening. "My name is Dr. Stephen Seager. I'm a psychiatrist at Benjamin Miller Hospital. John Doe was a patient of mine. Someone needs to contact his relatives."

"Why didn't you say so, Doc?" the woman said, reversing her tone. "You wouldn't believe the goofy calls we get down here. We try to screen them. Let me ring Dr. Rodriguez for you. He might be able to help." While she waited for the pathologist to answer, the woman made polite conversation.

"So this Doe was a loon, huh?" she said airily.

"Pardon me?"

"Still, even someone like that deserves better," the woman continued.

"'Someone' as in a normal human being, you mean?" was what I wanted to say but the other doctor came on the line. Dr. Rodriguez seemed startled to have anyone calling him. I asked about John Doe.

"We can't come up with a name either," Rodriguez said. "But we don't have the resources to look very hard. Unless someone claims the remains, there's not much else to be done. There are so many of these people."

I said I understood then asked a question that wouldn't have occurred to me before talking with Bear. "What about burial arrangements?"

"It's a County contract," Rodriguez replied with a hitch in his voice. "We don't have control over that."

"I'll check back later to be sure." My voice had an uncharacteristic resolve.

"The plans will be seen to personally," Rodriguez replied.

I thanked the doctor, hung up then checked the clock on the wall. "Damn," I muttered, stuffing the phone number of the job placement service into a shirt pocket and heading for the elevator.

I was late for the ward "milieu" meeting. This was a weekly affair in which all the psychiatry staff gathered, ward and ER alike, to discuss any interpersonal problems we might be having with each other. Meant to correct misunderstandings while they were still small, before anything got out of hand, it was the one meeting in which patient care wasn't discussed.

The term "milieu" is derived from the work of Maxwell Jones an English psychiatrist during the 1940s. Toward the end of World War II, he was charged with caring for the returning English psychiatric casualties. He assembled a hospital staff.

As was the case with all the combatant nations, however, the number of mentally disabled veterans far outstripped any estimates. Jones and his group were quickly overwhelmed. There weren't enough doctors to go around. In a stroke of genius borne out of necessity, Jones decided to alter the definition of "doctor." He made each staff person on his wards a "therapist," all with a mutual say in every decision. Then he gave the same rights to his patients. Everyone was in the mix. He called this a "milieu."

Jones' approach solved the overcrowding problem nicely. The first thing for which everyone voted was to go home. And they did. His basic notion stuck, however, and forever altered the way psychiatric wards are structured. Our staff is a group of equals. We talk things over and work out difficulties together. It's a good idea.

When I walked into the conference room everyone else was already seated. Dupree, Hundley, Salazar, Townes, Tina and Yang were scattered among the nurses with Yates at one end of the table and, surprisingly, Bear at the other. Bear wasn't much for meetings. I took a seat. We knew what was on everyone's mind. There was no "Hello, girlfriend," from Yang.

A few minutes of painful small talk ensued before Yates, as was her manner, took control.

"We need to talk about John Doe," she said, as if checking an item off a list. We were all quiet.

"Damn shame," Yang said finally.

Salazar looked anguished.

"How could the court possibly release that guy?" Hundley added.

"Court's just following the law," Bear said.

"Who wrote the stupid law?" Dupree asked. Not many people around the table knew the answer.

"The state legislature," Bear said. "Our representatives. The people we voted for."

Yang perked. "I never voted for this mess—sick people living in the street."

"But you tolerate it," Bear stated directly at Yang. "You and me. We all do."

"There's a million people in the gutter or worse because they're ill," Bear continued. "And probably two-hundred thousand kids. Most of whom don't go to school." Then he sat back. "What will future generations think about us?"

"Not much," I said quietly.

"They'll think of us like we do slave owners in the old South," Bear said. "And they'll be right. We're not the first people to tolerate a moral disgrace, just the most recent."

Yates looked startled. "What can I do about any of this?"

"Who's your state legislator?" Bear replied.

Yates thought for a moment. "I'm not sure."

Again silence fell around the table. Only this time it was deep, almost palpable, like fog. At last, Tina pulled something from her pocket. "It's a sympathy card," she explained. "I thought we could all sign and send it to John Doe's relatives. He must have someone somewhere. I know it's probably silly."

"Not at all," I interrupted. "In fact, I've been thinking about sort of the same thing."

Bear appeared unsettled. The card made its way around the table. I wrote my name and passed it to him. He was last in line.

Bear fingered the card slowly, touching each corner. I didn't like the look on his face. He set the card on the table and stood. "Fuck it," he said and, finding the wall with his hand, headed for the door.

I exploded like a volcano. Everything with Linda, LA, John Doe, Jamal Johnson and sick people living in the sewer suddenly came bubbling to the surface.

"And fuck you, too!" I shouted. "We're just trying to do something decent. What the hell is the matter with you anyway?"

Bear stopped for a second. Without a word, his enormous frame disappeared out into the hall.

The staff's eyes were wide with astonishment. One attending physician screaming at another didn't happen every day, and certainly no one had ever gone after Bear.

"I'll be right back," I stuttered, snatching the card off the table.

"Good luck, girlfriend," Yang said.

"Mercy," Yates whispered.

I caught Bear just outside the locked ward door.

"Sorry," I said, touching his shoulder so he'd turn around. "I don't know what came over me."

"I know what came over you," Bear said, his face impassive. "It's what comes over all 'decent folks' when a white person dies. Suddenly everything's a big fucking deal. We're having meetings and sending shit. Christ, a dozen black men have died out there since John Doe bought it. What about them?"

"I was just upset that you walked out of the meeting." We were on hot ground.

Bear took a breath and seemed to relax a bit. "The man's gone," he said slowly. "It's over. Enough's enough. No card, no nothin' is going to change that. Dying is what people do around here. Death is a growth industry in the ghetto. It's about the only thing you can count on."

"Do you know how many people were murdered on LA streets last year?" he asked and, actually, I did. I'd heard a piece about ghetto deaths on the radio but said nothing.

"Seven hundred," Bear stated, the emotion returning to his voice. "And lots of them were mentally ill like John Doe. Sorry, I can't stay worked up over one guy."

"I don't know about all seven hundred," I stammered. "But John Doe was our patient."

Bear ran a hand back across his head. "Give me the damn thing," he said reaching out his hand. I quickly slid the card to him and flicked open a pen. He took both and, using the wall for backing, felt for a blank spot on the open card then scribbled his name.

He gave me back the card and laughed. "Black man gets shot—nothing. White man drowns—look out."

I watched Bear walk away and get into the elevator. The doors slid closed. I looked down at the card, but not for long. There was a ruckus back on the ward. Chairs began crashing. Blows were being struck as screams rang out.

III

Running, I whipped out my keys then fumbled to unlock the door. All the while the shrieking continued. First trying my car key then my house key, I finally happened upon the correct one, threw open the door and ran inside. In the hallway, a boxing match was going on. The two combatants fought in the center of a ring of staff people plastered against the walls in terror. Inside the nursing station, Yates was frantically dialing for the security police. No one wanted to step forward and stop the struggle. Nor, in fact, did I.

The woman was enormous. Her name was Lula Butts. Rumor had it that she'd once wrestled professionally. Lula, a ward "regular," had bipolar disorder. About four times a year she'd stop taking her meds, have a manic period and land in the hospital. She'd only been with us a little more than a week this time, so she was still "high."

The object of her wrath that morning was a frail black man, also a "frequent flyer" on the ward, whom we knew only as Rev. Ike. Rev. Ike was in his sixties and lived on the streets. He'd been a patient at the state hospital for many years but had been "de-institutionalized" back to the community. He claimed to be the pastor of the "The Living Jesus and Mary Church" but could never give us an address for the building nor a description of his congregation. But he did look the part. He always wore a long black cassock with a terribly stained but still recognizable white collar appropriately turned backwards. The fact that he'd written the word "HOWDY" on it did tend to detract somewhat from his ecclesiastical demeanor.

Lula had Rev. Ike by the scruff of his neck and was holding him at arm's length; the man's feet were barely touching the floor. "Keep still you little prick so I can hit you again," Lula boomed.

Rev. Ike danced and dodged at the end of Lula's arm like a puppet. Lula had her other hand gathered into an enormous ball and was aiming it at the bobbing marionette.

"Holy Jesus and his little lamb Mary," Rev. Ike mumbled over and over as he wiggled and squirmed to escape the certain doom awaiting him at the end of Lula's arm.

Yang, Hundley and Salazar were desperately glancing from side to side. Finally, they all looked at me. "Let's go!" I shouted and, in unison, we scrambled forward. Yang grabbed Rev. Ike and tried to pull him away but Lula wouldn't let go, so the poor man was now stretched horizontally in the air. Hundley began to pry at Lula's fingers, which were wrapped around Rev. Ike's throat. Salazar and I took hold of her free arm. In an effort to loosen her extremity, Lula began bouncing us up and down like children on a see-saw.

Lula could have launched the two of us at any moment and then mopped the floor with Yang and Hundley, but that didn't happen. Instead, the security officers arrived. It was, of course, the same group who'd come to rescue me from John Doe days before.

After some talking and a good show of force, Lula released Rev. Ike. He, Hundley and Yang stood in a panting knot as Salazar and I released her arm. She was taken to her room to cool down.

The security officers didn't say anything to me. As they led Lula away, however, two of them glanced back and shook their heads.

Bus Rides and Baseball Games

AS EVERYONE RETURNED TO WORK—we decided the milieu meeting was over—I stood for a moment in the hall looking at the sympathy card in my hand, now crumpled from the recent fracas. Smoothing out the wrinkles, I thought of John Doe and my conversation that morning with the coroner.

If I was ever going to find out about the man, it would have to be from someone who had known him. What better place to start than the patients on the floor? However briefly, they'd lived with him. John Doe must have said something to someone, sometime.

Lula was the best person with whom to begin. Despite her outburst that morning, she was, once medicated, a sweet woman. Other patients gravitated to her. If John Doe had revealed anything, it would have been to Lula.

That evening she was much calmer. I found her in the ward day room, her huge body engulfing a chair. Ironically, Rev. Ike was sitting beside her. They were watching *Jeopardy*.

"Bolivia!" Lula shouted. She was better but not well. She nudged Rev. Ike. "Any fool knows that. I've watched this show for ten years. Asked the same question in '88. Damn, gotta get on that program."

"Bless Jesus and his little lamb Mary," Rev. Ike muttered.

"Mind if I join you?" I asked, pulling up a chair.

"Dr. Seager! Come on, sit down. It's Bolivia, you know, Sucre and La Paz," Lula said, smiling broadly and pointing to Alex Trebek. "Country with two capitals. Also Laos—Vientiane and Luang Probang. But that wasn't part of the question. South Africa has three."

Lula's fund of knowledge was impressive. She was, as the final *Jeopardy* answer proved, correct. Two computer scientists got the answer wrong.

Touching her arm, I redirected Lula's attention. "I've got a problem. Maybe you and Reverend Ike can help me."

"Anything, Baby," Lula cooed seductively. Hypersexuality was a symptom of her disease.

"Praise Jesus and his little lamb Mary," Rev. Ike said and leaned in closer.

"I want to find out more about John Doe," I began. "You remember. He was up here on the ward. Got released by the court."

Lula nodded. "Strange bird. Hear he got drowned. Too bad."

"That's the one."

"Why do you want to know about him?" she asked.

That was a difficult question to answer. "We've got a sympathy card for his family that the staff all signed. I'd like to find out where he lived. He told the judge he had a place on 39th and Crenshaw."

Rev. Ike and Lula looked at each other. At last Lula spoke. "He didn't say nothin' about that to me. We all figured the fella didn't live anywhere. There are thousands of crazies like him out there. They don't stay no place. They're just...around."

Rev. Ike nodded. "Praise Jesus and his little lamb Mary," he commented.

"Is there anything you know that might help me?" I persisted.

Lula thought for a moment. "He said something once about the Number 14 bus. That's about it."

"Great, does the Number 14 go by 39th street?"

"Yeah," Lula said. "It runs down Crenshaw right past there. Mainly, though, it just winds through the neighborhood then heads Downtown toward Skid Row. You aren't thinking of gettin' on that thing, are you?"

"Why?" I tried to sound nonchalant.

"Nobody rides that bus," Lula continued and Rev. Ike agreed, nodding again. "Too dangerous. Best you get any idea like that out of your head."

I drooped into my seat, disappointed. "Thanks anyway."

"You take things too personal," Lula said, patting my knee. "John Doe's gone. We all feel bad. But, shit, the man's dead. That kinda stuff happens every day."

II

For the next week, concentrating on work was nearly impossible. John Doe was stuck in my mind. I frequently found myself opening the top drawer of my desk to look at his sympathy card, and my thoughts would drift back to Lula's comment about the Number 14 bus. I tried to imagine who was riding it and where they were going. Attempting to conjure up an image of 39th and Crenshaw, I went over its route a thousand times.

The Number 14 bus began to haunt me. Every time I walked out-side it seemed to be rolling by, thick exhaust billowing behind in dark, noxious blasts. When I crossed the street, it was at the corner. Turning to the squeal of brakes, there was the Number 14 expelling one group of riders and accepting another. I even began to dream about it.

I had unfinished business with John Doe, and the Number 14 was his bus. Somewhere along its convoluted trail, hopefully at 39th and Crenshaw, was his home and my only chance of discovering who he really was.

Wednesday, around noon, as I was heading to lunch, the Num-ber 14 bus stopped in front of the hospital. The suspense was intoler-able. I had an appointment with Tina, Dupree and Yang at three. There was time.

Surprisingly, it wasn't all that traumatic. Fishing a dollar from my pocket and waving to the driver, I hopped on board, walked down the aisle and took a seat.

The man beside me was wearing a foul-smelling trench coat. But that wasn't what caught my interest. It was the do-it-yourself alumi-num foil space helmet on his head. He noticed me staring.

"Keeps out any brain-sapping rays," the man whispered, point-ing to the sky. "From the Planet Drano."

Angling over a bit, I peered out the window. "They can be murder this time of day," I said. Nodding, the man hunched down as the bus suddenly lurched forward.

It was difficult sorting out my emotions as we rumbled haltingly down Rosecrans Boulevard then turned left on Crenshaw. I was scared to death. The urge to scream and run was unexpectedly powerful. The depth of that fear startled and confused me. After years of training at County General, I imagined that I'd come to grips with the ghetto, that we had some kind of mutual understanding. The bus hadn't gone ten blocks, however, before I realized how wrong that was.

What I did know about the ghetto was where the best lit roads in and out were, how it looked nine to five on weekdays from my office window and the two-block walk from the Mill to McDonald's. Despite my supposed experience, I'd never actually been *in* the ghetto, never really come to know it firsthand.

I was scared, and not simply from sitting alone in a sea of black faces; it was more visceral than that. The place felt so alien. It was as if we were touring another country, one where I didn't know the people, language or rules. What frightened me most was that there actually might not be any rules. The fact that seven hundred people had been murdered in LA over the last year finally meant something. If a fellow rider were to suddenly stand and shoot me dead, the other people would have been startled but not surprised. I was traveling through a place where, "Call the police," would probably have stirred only minor interest.

After I'd calmed down a bit, the bus pulled to a stop at the 39th street intersection. We were there. Still battling my nerves, I looked outside. Nothing. All four corner lots were empty, apparently bulldozed to the ground. Clearly, John Doe hadn't lived here. There wasn't any abandoned building and certainly no "reputable" restaurants.

Distraught, I found enough courage to speak to a woman two seats behind me. "Has the corner always been like this?"

She glanced out the window. "Since '84," she said. "For the Olympics. The Man came in and took down lots of rundown places. Didn't want the world to think bad of us. Used the government money to redo the airport. Left this behind."

I was appalled but said nothing.

As the bus eased away, I recalled what Lula had said: "Those guys don't live nowhere. They're just around." As bad as this place was—block after endless block of dilapidated homes, open drain pipes, rusted fences, ill-fed children and garbage-strewn streets—I knew that in order to discover anything about John Doe it meant going even deeper than the ghetto. There was yet another still more desolate layer of the city to be uncovered, the subterranean world of the homeless mentally ill. The ghetto was bad enough but this other place had to be worse.

If I wanted to deliver the sympathy card, however, I had to ride the bus further then actually get off. But it wouldn't be that day. I was too unnerved. Glued to my seat like a statue, my thoughts were in disarray. I would see this ride through to the finish, and that was it. I'd had enough disappointment for one day.

After our initial conversation, the man in the aluminum hat didn't speak again nor did he pull his head from the protective cocoon of jacked-up coat lapels. He must have been running on some kind of internal timer or secretly counting the stops because he suddenly leapt up and darted off the bus. Maybe he'd exited at random, when the rays finally became unbearable.

Three other people sat next to me during the trip: an older black gentleman in a meticulously brushed and blocked felt hat, a middle-aged woman who kept a paper bag firmly planted in her lap and, tragically, a young Hispanic girl of no more than fifteen. Her hair was tangled. She wore three layers of dirty clothes. Her face was bruised on one side—all telltale marks of life on the streets. She, too, seemed to leave the bus haphazardly. I didn't say anything to any of them. In retrospect, I should have spoken to the girl, given her money or the address of the hospital. Or something.

At least one thing could be said for the Number 14 bus: it ran on time. We chugged through the ghetto, drove around Downtown and arrived back at the Mill two hours later, on the dot.

"Enjoy the show?" the burly driver said as I stood to leave. I couldn't think of anything to say.

I was never so glad to see the Mill in all my life. It may have been a somewhat rundown building in a bad neighborhood, but it was my rundown building in my bad neighborhood. Besides, my car was there. The car that would take me home.

A few days passed before I could look at the Number 14 bus again. But it was still there, going by every two hours like clockwork. And John Doe's card was in my desk, egging me, taunting me into further action.

III

The immediate future had nothing to do with either the Number 14 bus or John Doe. Instead, a baseball game at Dodger stadium, an outing for our patients who were doing well, was on the agenda. The ward staff would chaperone this activity, part of a new County program, which, in these days of shrinking budgets, was a welcome change.

The intent was for our patients to develop more "real world" skills by putting them in situations where previously they might have had trouble. With support, instruction and guidance, these obstacles might be conquered. It also gave us a chance to measure our patients' progress outside the artificial confines of the ward.

The selection of a baseball game for the excursion hadn't been easy. All interested staff and selected patients had gathered in the ward conference room—a seemingly banal event—to confirm our destination.

Tina, Hundley, Yang, Yates and myself represented the staff. Six patients were there. Yates began with a precise explanation of the rules; a mutually acceptable location would be chosen, and everyone had a vote. The floor was then opened for suggestions.

First to speak was Luther Alexander, a middle-aged former insurance executive now tormented by recurrent bouts of severe depression. "We should go to a strip club. 'Bare Elegance' is nice," he said with a broad smile, a sign that he was almost ready to go home.

When Yates bristled, two other patients, Norman Colter and Ted Green, both just coming down from manic swings, flew into action.

"Strip club's a good idea," Colter concurred. "It could be very educational. Learning how to make change, give tips and all."

"There is absolutely no way..." Yates began to rise from her chair, but Green beat her to the punch.

"I agree with Colter," he spouted. "It's our trip. You said we could go where we wanted."

"Shit, fuck, piss. Sorry," added Carlos Villegas. "Strip clubs are great."

Carlos suffered from Tourette's syndrome; compulsive swearing was one of his symptoms. His disease had been under control, but this recent burst of excitement seemed to have fostered a momentary regression.

The staff eyed one another nervously. Things were getting out of hand.

"We're going to a baseball game," Lula finally said, coming to our rescue, edging forward in her seat to emphasize the finality of this decision. She winked at me. "Gotta see all those cute boys in their tight pants."

Everyone looked at Lula. Then at each other.

"Baseball game is fine," Alexander said.

"National pastime," echoed Colter, his eyes never leaving Lula's massive arms.

"Okay by me," agreed Green.

"Baseball, piss yes," said Carlos.

"Praise Jesus and his little lamb Mary," concluded Rev. Ike.

IV

I was grateful for Lula's idea. Baseball is in my blood. There's nothing I enjoy more than a night at the ballpark. My fondest memory from childhood was my ten-year-old Little League baseball team winning the Ogden City Championship. After the game, during a celebratory melee, my hat got thrown in the air, landing at the top of a nearby tree where, as far as I know, it remains today.

However, I had mixed feelings about that particular game. Traveling out into the community with patients was a new idea. Who knew what could happen?

The County van arrived at six P.M., pulling to the curb in front of the Mill. Yang had taken up a collection during the week so that, in addition to ticket money, there was cash for hot dogs and sodas. Before leaving, we did a quick head count and distributed the funds.

I was a little nervous about Carlos. "How are you feeling?" I ventured tentatively.

There was a pause. "Fine, I guess," he said at last.

"That's good." A cheerful tone concealed my concern.

All the patients filed into the vehicle until only Lula was left. She wasn't going through the van door. Not that she didn't try; she was simply too large. It was an unexpected problem. With no other alternative, Lula put one foot inside as Yang, Hundley and I got behind her.

"Sorry, Lula," I said as we placed our hands on either side of her mammoth rear end.

"Pleasure's all mine," Lula grinned, and everyone laughed. With a lot of pushing, some tucking and finally the use of Hundley's shoulder, she was in. The rest of us climbed aboard, and we were off.

Everyone immediately began to chatter. Listening to their conversations, I surmised from my seat in the back that this collection of people was many things but not, apparently, big sports fans.

"Will there be a half-time show?" Crystal Adams, a wispish, recovering schizophrenic, asked as we eased onto the Harbor Freeway.

"Honey, there's no half-time in baseball," Colter answered. "That's only in hockey."

Struggling to turn her massive frame, Lula looked at Colter and Adams then rolled her eyes. "Lord, give me strength," she muttered.

The discussions continued. Yang spoke with Tina who sat beside him near the driver. Colter and Green pointed out the passing sights. Hundley and I were keeping our fingers crossed. Carlos and Rev. Ike, positioned beside us, were both silent, eyes straight ahead. Luther Alexander and Yates were a row up. Surprisingly, they were engrossed in conversation. Every so often I heard Yates giggle, which was definitely something new.

After parking the van and traversing the asphalt lot, the group joined a line to buy tickets. After the staff was taken care of, Lula then Colter, Green, Adams, Alexander and Rev. Ike paid their money, received their change and left the ticket booth without a hitch. Only Carlos remained. Yang and I were standing beside him, just in case.

"One, please. Right field pavilion," Carlos said, handing a ten dollar bill to the crisp, smiling young woman behind the counter.

She, still smiling, gave Carlos his change. "Thanks, bitch," Carlos blurted, his face dropping.

"I beg your pardon?" the woman sputtered. She'd stopped smiling.

"You cock-sucking, nigger, whore!" Carlos shouted, the terror building in his eyes. He pounded both fists on the counter in frustration. It sounded like rifle fire.

"Security!" the woman screamed, standing bolt straight.

Yang and I grabbed Carlos' change and his ticket, then I pushed the man toward Yang who yanked him forward.

"He has a disease," I said quickly to the now trembling young woman. Her Dodger hat was atilt. "He's on medication. He can't help it."

"Why don't you take that jerk to a doctor?!" the woman shouted as Yang, Hundley, Tina, Yates and I tried to hustle everyone quickly toward the stadium gate.

"We are doctors," I called out.

"Well, you're pretty damn poor then," the woman retorted in a final salvo. Near the entrance, I turned and looked back. The other people in line were staring. In the distance, a blue uniformed guard was striding toward the ticket booth.

"No sweat, Carlos, you did fine," I reassured him once we were safely inside the park.

Carlos seemed visibly relieved. "Thanks, asshole," he murmured.

The evening proceeded, unfortunately, as it had begun. Green and Colter sneaked a few beers, eventually striking up a shouting match with an equally drunken man four rows over. Then they got into it with Yates who, by the fifth inning, was livid. Yang and Tina discussed modern dance and opera, oblivious to anything happening on the field. Crystal Adams wandered off, and it took Hundley an hour to find her. Then there was Lula. She flirted so shamelessly with the Dodger rightfielder, Hundley and I had to calm her down before someone stopped the game.

Mercifully, we got involved with the stadium police only once. Spotting them escorting Carlos out of the men's bathroom, I slapped Hundley's shoulder. We jumped up so quickly I spilled a large Coke onto the shoes of the fans sitting in front of me. I didn't ask what Carlos had said. It was all we could do to keep the cops from arresting him. I explained that he was sick. Hundley and I had to show our hospital I.D.s.

Only Rev. Ike remained blissfully unperturbed. "Praise Jesus and His little lamb Mary," he said to a hot dog vendor.

"Amen," the man replied, surveying the group.

Mercifully, the game was over quickly. Mike Piazza, the Dodger catcher, hit a home run in the bottom of the eighth inning and the home team prevailed 3–1.

"That was fun," Carlos said as we boarded the van to head home.

"Give it a rest," Yates sighed, crumpling into the back seat. Exhausted, I sat beside her after, once again, shoehorning Lula back inside the vehicle.

Drained from their night of social conquest, the patients all dozed on the way home. After a bit, I too let my eyelids close, blissfully unaware of what lay ahead.

Epiphany on Skid Row

THE REMAINDER OF THE WEEKEND PASSED UNEVENT-
FULLY. Linda was on edge but allowed herself to be comforted by my
assurance that I'd already begun looking for another job. I comforted myself by saying that definitely was my plan.

Driving to work on Monday, I was again thinking about the
Number 14 bus and the sympathy card in my desk drawer. I pulled
into the parking lot and walked past the psych ER on my way upstairs
for rounds. I never made it.

Bull and Ten-Trees were standing outside in the lobby. They motioned me over. "What's up?" I asked.

"Someone's here to see you," Bull said, opening the ER door.

Once inside, I stopped in my tracks. I'd totally forgotten. In the
first room across from the nursing station, fumbling through a
drawer filled with tongue depressors, was Jamal Johnson. He was
alone.

"Grandma Naomi's real sick. She's on the seventh floor," Jamal
stammered while whipping the drawer closed. "The doctors say it's
her heart. She sent me to wait for you."

"Let's go," I said, ushering the boy out of the room. Neither of us
spoke as I walked and he ran down the hallway to the main hospital
elevators. Riding up seven flights, fighting tears, Jamal fidgeted the
whole way.

As we neared the intensive care unit, I had an increasingly un-
comfortable feeling. As a medical doctor, the ICU had been a routine
part of my life. But I'd never come to one like this, a visitor with a
lump in my throat.

I hesitantly left Jamal in a small waiting area and headed through the doors. It took me a second to absorb the place, all the tubes, machines, blinking lights and alarms beeping. The sheer volume of technology required to battle death always astounded me. Then I saw Naomi Johnson lying in bed three.

Walking over, my legs felt wobbly. I took hold of a side rail just in case. Hooked to a heart monitor and IV lines, Naomi looked so frail. I'd seen people like this many times. Her breathing was labored. Fluid was rapidly accumulating in her lungs. She was going to die.

She opened her eyes and, through everything, managed a smile. "So glad...to see...you," she whispered and took my hand.

"I wish it didn't have to..." I began but Naomi shook her head.

"There's... no time," she puffed. "I've...got everything... you'll...need." Her breath was coming harder by the second. She gestured toward a nightstand upon which Jamal's records and a frayed family Bible lay.

I touched the mound of papers: immunization records, psychological tests, X-ray reports, school summaries, etc., everything Naomi had been able to gather, documenting in minute detail, the short but chaotic life of her only grandson. I riffled a worn corner of the Bible, then Naomi gently squeezed my fingers.

"God bless you," she said in a feather-light voice and closed her eyes.

Instantly, the bedside heart monitor let out a piercing, sustained whistle, and the line on the screen went flat. Pandemonium erupted. People were running everywhere. "CODE BLUE, ICU. CODE BLUE, ICU," the overhead operator stated repeatedly. The doors burst open, and a phalanx of white coats came running in.

Grabbing Naomi's effects and edging away, I let the resuscitation team do its job. Eventually, she was no longer visible, her bed engulfed with frantic people.

After a few minutes, Ms. Carlson, one of the unit nurses, caught my attention. While the battle to save Naomi raged on, Carlson was tending to the central monitor station, watching the other patients' vital signs. "Friend?" she asked.

"Her grandson's a patient of mine."

Carlson glanced toward bed three. "She's quite a woman."

"You're right."

"A real fighter," she said admiringly. "She should have died last night. It's like she was holding out. Waiting for something."

I tucked Naomi's things under my arm, then went to sit with Jamal in the waiting room. He'd scattered every magazine in the place and was fumbling with the window lock. I took a seat—we were the only ones there—and let him roam. After fifteen minutes, Carlson got my attention from the door. She shook her head.

"It's over," I said, turning to Jamal. "Your grandmother's dead."

Across the room, he stopped in his tracks. His bottom lip began to tremble. "What happens to me now?"

I walked over and pulled him close. "I don't know."

"You won't send me back to my mother, will you?" Jamal asked, twitching beneath my arm.

"We'll do our best to see that doesn't happen. I promised Naomi. Now I'm promising you."

Jamal could no longer contain his emotions, burying his head into my side. "Where will I go?" he sobbed.

"You'll stay at a foster home until things get straightened out." I held the boy tight. "But I won't leave or forget you."

After a while Jamal quieted down a bit. As if playing a bass drum, only his foot was tapping regularly. I left the waiting room to call the County children's service people, explained the situation, then went in again to sit with Jamal. By then he'd begun to pace. Within the hour, a woman came to pick him up. He warily took her hand, looking back at me from the waiting room door. "I promise," I said. As the pair left, Jamal impulsively snatched two pens from a small tabletop and stuck them in his pocket.

II

The rest of the day is mostly a blur. I took care of business on the ward then, late in the afternoon, stopped by my office. Naomi's Bible and papers were on top of the desk. Pulling out a chair, I sat, propping my feet on the window ledge. I don't remember leaving to go home or what happened that night.

The following day was our shift in the psych ER. Trying to put Jamal out of my mind, from morning until 4:30, Tina, Yang, Dupree and I plowed through the usual collection of sick people who'd meandered into traffic, attacked someone, been attacked or disrupted commerce at local stores. We sedated crackheads and speed users, lost in the depths of drug-induced psychotic spirals. We saw a depressed school teacher, a suicidal teen and talked to a few souls who simply needed somewhere to rest for a while.

That evening I took Mike and Jake to the park and hit ground balls to them. Afterwards, we went for a soda. It occupied some time. At dusk, we headed home. After dinner and a cable movie, Linda went to bed. I didn't mention Naomi.

The next morning, at a stoplight near the hospital, the Number 14 bus rolled through the intersection in front of me and sputtered down the road. I did my best to ignore the smoking behemoth, accelerating away as the light turned.

John Doe was again on my mind as I walked onto the ward before morning rounds. Remembering a loose end, I stopped in the nursing station to phone Dr. Rodriguez at the County morgue. "Mr. Doe was buried a week ago," Rodriguez told me. "Saw to it myself."

"Why didn't you call? We wanted to be there."

Rodriguez paused. "Forgive me," he said at last. "In all my years, that's never happened."

A family's son was dead and buried, and they didn't know about it. This steeled my resolve to track down John Doe's identity, and my game plan began to rapidly formalize. In retrospect, I should have thought things out a little more thoroughly.

III

I didn't dare tell anyone what I was thinking, which should have been a clue that my scheme probably wouldn't work. In turmoil about Jamal, about Linda and my job, my judgment was off. But my mind was made up. I had a sympathy card to deliver.

After hurrying through the day's work and following a late lunch, I went to my office and took John Doe's card from the desk drawer. Momentarily setting my keys and wallet on the chair, I opened the card and read it again. I thought of John Doe's parents, and my stomach hurt. Sliding the card into a back pocket, I checked the time. "Shit," I mumbled, snatching enough change for the bus from a small dish on my desk and heading out. It was already getting late. I was wearing my favorite red shirt, pocket out.

"Family situation, nothing serious," I told Candy, the clerk at the front desk. "Probably won't be back today."

As always, the Number 14 bus appeared on schedule, and this time I boarded with somewhat less trepidation. Taking a seat behind the driver, we'd only gone a few blocks before I decided to get down to business. Leaning forward, I began timidly. "Excuse me. This may sound strange, but I'm trying to track down the identity of a homeless mentally ill man. He died, and the family needs to be notified." The driver kept his eyes forward. "He rode this bus," I persisted. "Used the name John Doe. A white guy about twenty-five. Chronic schizophrenic. Called everyone Nazis." My voice trailed off. The driver was ignoring me. He took one hand off the wheel and pointed to a small sign in the middle of the dash.

"Do Not Speak To Driver While Bus Is In Motion," it read.

"Sorry," I said and sat back.

As the bus swayed and rocked along, stopping and starting while dozens of faceless people got off and other faceless people got on, the utter futility of my venture began to sink in. The ghetto seemed to go on forever. I was looking for a needle in a haystack of disaster.

We'd been riding for thirty minutes when the bus finally left the ghetto, ruled by crack cocaine, and entered Skid Row, the world of alcoholics. The driver pulled to the curb beside a seedy tavern at the corner of two dreary, dismal streets. Depressed but determined, I thought this was as good a place as any to start and stood to leave. The driver, however, now checking traffic in his side mirror, reached out and shook his hand as if to say, "not here."

Confused but excited I sat down again. Apparently, he'd heard me after all. My waning spirits began to rise.

After another mile, we stopped in the middle of a block, something new, in front of a small, seemingly abandoned warehouse. A bullet-pocked, weathered sign hung above two large wooden doors: "Safe Haven Rescue Mission."

The bus doors whooshed open, and the driver finally spoke. "Ask for Big John," he said, without turning. "And God help you."

I don't recall thanking him because, the instant I stepped off the bus, I was surrounded.

"Spare change?" said a man with a "ZZ Top" beard and shoulder-to-shoulder tattoos, gruffly thrusting a hand toward me.

"Nice shirt," an even stragglier fellow lisped, fingering the cloth of my left sleeve. He had no teeth.

"Got money for food?" demanded a third person, reeking of gin. He was swaying two inches from my face.

It was time to scream and run. Turning to hail the bus, its exhaust trail was just fading around the corner. Certain the three men were going to stab me, I almost wet my pants.

Then, like Daniel in the lion's den, I was saved. The front doors of the mission exploded open and Goliath himself stood in the maw. "Dinner!" he shouted, and with that my tormentors were gone, scrambling to join an instantly assembled line of people forming at the entrance. They came from alleyways, behind dumpsters and out of rusting, tire-less cars slumped at the curb. They sprang, it seemed, from the very refuse that lay rotting in the gutter.

Watching this, I was filled with the strangest sense of nauseating familiarity. There were men in that queue so filthy their skin was no longer visible and women so rank with accumulated secretions even the dirt-stained men turned away. Children were gaunt from malnutrition. Nearly everyone had either open sores, poorly healed fractures or caked blood. I could see the lice and vermin. They were a symphony of coughs and wheezes.

"Are you new to the streets?" the enormous man asked, approaching me as the food line continued to grow.

"Pardon?" I queried, not certain I'd heard right.

"You're new to the streets, right?" he said in a voice incongruously compassionate with his oak-tree frame. Dressed in a plaid shirt, khaki pants and sporting an enormous red beard, he looked like Paul Bunyan.

"You must be Big John. I was told to ask for you."

"Join us for dinner," Big John commanded, draping a bulky arm around my shoulder and turning me toward the shelter doorway.

"No, that's not it," I protested, feeling more angry than the situation warranted. "I'm looking for someone."

"Aren't we all," Big John said laughing out loud. "Don't worry. The first time's always the worst. Sharp fella like you, though, you'll be back on your feet in no time."

"No, no," I insisted, still bucking Big John's pull. "Let me show you my ID." Stopping, I reached back and extracted John Doe's sympathy card. Panic stricken, I slapped my other hip. Then fished in my shirt pocket. Nothing. The image of my wallet and keys sitting on the desk chair came to me. "For God's sake," I muttered, jabbing into my pockets again.

"Whoever you are," Big John said, turning to gauge the slant of the afternoon light. "If you want to eat, it better be soon. Things have to be wrapped up by sunset."

I checked my watch. It was already past four, and I hadn't even begun to search for information about John Doe.

"My name is Dr. Seager," I said. "I'm a psychiatrist at Benjamin Miller Medical Center, and I'm trying to track down the last whereabouts of a patient. The man died, and his family should know. He went by the name of John Doe."

Big John cast me an understanding glance, the look of a man who'd heard all the stories before and had long ago given up trying to decide which ones were true. I knew this expression well. I used it on patients in the psych ER frequently.

"Start with the flophouse hotels," Big John said, starting to walk back toward the mission. "But remember, when it's dark, dinner's over, the doors are locked."

A recent arrival, scurrying toward the food line, abruptly stopped beside me. He couldn't have been more than nineteen. There was a wad of chewing gum in his hair. "Spare change?" he asked mechanically.

"Go away," I barked. Fifteen minutes on the streets, and already I'd begun to harden.

IV

Heading away from the mission, I walked two blocks down a nearby side street. The number of decaying, rat-infested buildings that passed for "hotels" astounded me. There was almost nothing else.

I chose one at random, a two-story affair with missing window-panes and a sign that read "The Palms." There wasn't a tree in sight. The tubercular counter man said he'd never heard of John Doe. I checked a second hotel, a third and then three dozen more. They all looked alike, each with equally ridiculous names. My experience at every place was the same; a grizzled man behind an unvarnished counter would glare when asked about John Doe, then reply, "Don't know anybody. If you want a room that'll be ten bucks."

I missed a few spots because either the clerks were nowhere to be found or were too drunk to wake. It was now 5:30. "What the hell am I doing here?" I said out loud, standing near the curb, tired and depressed.

Fortunately, there was still time to catch the Number 14 back to the hospital, return home before Linda became worried and get a desperately needed drink while soaking in a long bath.

Retracing my steps along the littered sidewalk, I finally saw the mission at a far corner. With a mild sense of elation, I hurried further down the street, looking for my ride back, the bus that would remove me from this mess. Instead, a thin column of black smoke appeared, wafting silently above the drab horizon.

V

Then there was a second smudgy plume. And a third. Inside of five minutes there were too many to count. "What the...?" I muttered. It was as if the entire city had instantaneously caught fire. Some of the blazes were nearby; the air quickly became acrid and difficult to breathe.

As I stood, flabbergasted, a few more people scuffled into the shelter. Then Big John burst through the doors again. He stopped, scanning the area for stragglers.

"Let's go!" he shouted, waving his hand.

I stumbled over, my eyes riveted on the ever blackening sky. "What's happening?" I stuttered.

"It just came over the radio. The King verdict's in. All four cops were acquitted. The city's exploding."

Now I was doubly confused. "Acquitted? How can that be?"

"Don't know," Big John said, pushing me the final few feet inside. "But we'll be lucky if they don't torch this place tonight with all of us in it."

"I've got to get home," I protested as Big John slid a bolt lock closed.

"Don't we all."

"But the bus..."

Big John shook his head. "That thing's probably been rolled and gutted by now. There'll be no way out of here tonight."

"Is there a phone?"

Big John pointed. "Pay phone on the wall."

I made a beeline across the shelter. Cradling the receiver between my shoulder and ear, I dug into my pants pockets producing one paper clip and a plastic pen top.

I turned and searched the room for Big John, who was suddenly nowhere in sight, while scouring both front pockets again right down to the lint.

Desperate, I quickly looked around the shelter crowd of one hundred or so trying to locate the most normal-looking person. He was a man in his thirties, wearing a sweatshirt and jeans. Hair combed and face deeply tanned, he looked like a construction worker. Walking over I fantasized that maybe he was also trapped here by some bizarre but explainable circumstance. I hoped he was one of "us," not one of "them."

"Excuse me," I began. The man was seated at the end of a bench behind a picnic-style table, of which there were ten in the room. Just beginning his meal, he didn't look up from his plate as I spoke. "Excuse me," I repeated in an embarrassed tone. "I need to make a phone call and my wallet..." was as far as I got before the man grabbed a plastic knife and whipped his head around. "I am the King. I can do anything," he seethed. "Carving eyes is my specialty."

My heart pounding like a trip-hammer, I could barely form words. "You're right. You're right," I mumbled over and over again, backing away from that knife.

An overwhelming desire to run engulfed me. Despite the fires and turmoil outside, I scrambled to the door, pulled the bolt open and dashed out. The evening sky was aglow with red. The air was soot and syrup. Distant shouts and the squeal of racing tires had replaced the city's normal emanations.

Standing on the sidewalk, I jumped as a low-rider car, headlights off and drunken occupants laughing, roared up. An arm reached out a back window and fired a gun, the bullet carving a chip from the pavement three feet to my right. Then the car zoomed away.

I was too stunned to move. Suddenly realizing the car might return, however, I pulled myself together enough to make it back into the shelter.

VI

I stood just inside the door, trying to sort out my predicament. The three men who'd accosted me on the sidewalk were glaring. Averting my gaze, I stared down at the floor. A roach the size of a quarter crawled across my shoe. At long last, I looked up just as Big John reappeared toward the back of the room. Time had come for a different tack.

"It doesn't matter who I am," I said, wending between tables and getting the man's attention. "What's important is making a phone call, and I don't have any money."

A broad, comforting smile passed across Big John's face. "Why didn't you say so?" He reached inside his shirt pocket, pulled out a quarter and handed it to me. "Gotta check in with the answering service, huh, Doc?"

"Yeah," I replied, clutching the coin like a drowning man grips a life jacket.

Unable to imagine what Linda and the boys might be thinking, I was at the phone again. Dropping the quarter into the money slot, I hurriedly punched in my home number, waiting one second, five and finally ten. The line was dead.

I slammed the receiver back into its cradle so hard the phone nearly ripped from the wall. A dozen people eating at the long tables momentarily looked up. Embarrassed and frustrated, I leaned against the wall.

As I gradually settled down, my adrenaline levels finally decreasing to somewhere near normal, I gazed out over the motley crowd ravenously devouring its dinner. Looking from face to face, I examined those who would spend the night and, judging from the tumult outside, perhaps many nights. Why were they here?

Some people glanced back but only momentarily. It took me a while to sort through my thoughts. These weren't just "street people" or "the homeless mentally ill." Each one was someone's child, brother, friend, sister, nephew, niece or parent. They hadn't always been here, always lived like this. These folks had all once belonged somewhere, been part of something, had people who loved them, people who worried about them. Then they'd become sick. They were all John Does.

Amazingly, I also realized that most of them were familiar to me. Not personally, perhaps, but in the sense that I could have diagnosed each one, explaining which neurotransmitters weren't functioning

properly in his or her brain. I could have accurately detailed everything recent research had to say about structural abnormalities in
their gray matter, which medications each person needed, what side
effects they might suffer and how long they could expect to live.
These were all things I'd learned from research papers, medical
school and during residency. The data. The facts and figures.

Now this wasn't enough. More questions than answers were going through my head. Despite years of study about mental illness, I
didn't really know much about the mentally ill at all. The diseases
were familiar to me but not the people. I only had a partial image of
who they were or what they were feeling. Were they as frightened as
I? Or had the constancy of havoc and chaos in their lives somehow
inured them to anarchy? How did they tolerate the squalor? The in-
festations? The insanity? The pain? Everything was absolutely still
for a second. It was a defining moment. "My God, what have we
done to these people?" I whispered to myself.

Everything was suddenly very clear. The reasons why mentally ill
people had to live like this didn't matter. Whether this mass of suffering humanity had been deinstitutionalized or was there because of
public indifference, changing mental health policy or court decisions
wasn't relevant. It was simply wrong.

Equally importantly, I understood that nothing could ever be
done to help them until we, as a society, grasped that being homeless
and mentally ill isn't a medical or psychiatric problem. Civil rights
and personal freedom aren't the issues either. It's a moral question.
That the brain-diseased must exist on our streets and eat garbage is a
sin. Period.

I could never view the mentally ill in the old way again. Nor
would I see myself in the same way any more. All of us were locked
into a larger problem. Things had to change. I had to change.

Oblivious to my internal revelations, the others in the shelter
went on about their business. Big John began distributing worn blankets and coverless pillows; dinner tables were being folded and
stored in a large closet set into the far wall. Despite the bedlam
around us, everyone collected his or her bedding, found a clear spot
on the floor and began to settle in for the night.

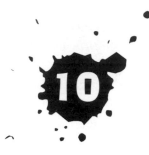

We Are Not the First

TO UNDERSTAND HOW WE'VE COME TO THIS STATE of near total neglect of the severely mentally ill, it's important to know their history. Twentieth century Americans aren't the first ones to misunderstand these people or treat them poorly. Throughout the years, others have struggled with different ideas about the cause of mental illness and what to do with those who suffer from it.

Two theories regarding the nature of brain disease emerged during ancient times and, unfortunately, have persisted in various forms to this day—mental disease as possession by evil spirits and insanity as punishment from God.

The priest class of Babylon and Nineva posited that the unusual behavior associated with mental illness was due to the work of demons. As such, the mentally ill were ostracized. Later, the Hebrews stated that mental disease occurred to those who weren't "right with God." It was a divine punishment for mortal transgression, so sick individuals were stoned to death.

In contrast, the Egyptians and Greeks got things right. Although believers in a magico-religious nature of mental illness, the ancient kings of Egypt didn't fear the brain diseased; they afforded treatment to them, building the first "asylums" designed for their care. Their approach was humane, including such things as boat trips on the Nile and musical concerts. Recreation therapy, teaching the mentally sick to create and enjoy, was invented there. We have rediscovered, in the twentieth century, the value of this modality; it's a cornerstone of modern in-hospital psychiatric care.

Greek medicine began with Aesculapius, a physician later my-thologized as the Roman god of healing, who built shrines for curing the sick, including the mentally ill. Emphasizing cleanliness, diet and rest, the temple doctors' ministrations also included a drug-induced "incubation" sleep during which snakes were produced from inside the caregivers' garments. The wiggling creatures would then lick the patients' feet. For unknown reasons, this was thought to be thera-peutic. Interestingly, the emblem of these early Greek sanitariums, the rod of Aesculapius with an entwined serpent, remains the symbol of medicine to this day.

Soon after Aesculapius, a complete shift in the way we view the universe occurred. As a means of explaining physical phenomena, the Greeks brought formalized logic and reasoning into existence. They were, in fact, the first people to conclude that the world actually *could* be understood.

Hippocrates of Cos applied these principles to illness, stating that sickness, whether mental or physical, was caused by identifiable, natural processes. For this he is known as the Father of Modern Medicine.

He classified the mental disorders as follows—delirium, epilepsy, mania, depression and paranoia—stating that these maladies resulted from a maldistribution of the body's "humors" or fluids. If you sub-stitute the word "neurotransmitter" for "humors," his theory correlates well with the current notion that mental illness is caused by a chemi-cal imbalance in the brain. Correcting this disparity is the proposed mechanism by which most present-day psychiatric drugs act.

Ironically, despite their tremendous intellectual advances, one root of our current mental health crisis can also be traced to the an-cient Greeks, back to a philosophical conflict between Plato and Ar-istotle. Plato espoused "didactic" reasoning, an approach which states that by applying the inviolate rules of logic and mathematics to a problem the true answer can invariably be derived. No experience or testing was necessary. We have an aphorism that summarizes this method: "It looks good on paper."

Aristotle refuted this model and introduced the concept of "em-piricism" or analytic reasoning. He said that personal experience and testing must be included in any final equation. In other words, according to Aristotle, what looks good on paper must also work in reality before we can label it as "true." As we shall see later, this theoretical clash had a profound effect on the course of modern American mental health policy.

After the decline of Greek civilization, the Roman empire flowered, and with it came new ideas concerning mental disease and its treatment. A series of philosophers addressed these issues in their writing. Aetaeus, in his first century book, *De Causis et Signis Morborum*, observed that manic and depressive states could occur in the same individual, with perfectly lucid intervals in between. This description of bipolar disease is erroneously attributed to Emil Kraeplin, the nineteenth century German giant of psychiatry.

Largus, in 4 B.C., was known to have experimented with electricity, Benjamin Franklin notwithstanding. Postulating that the mystical current originating from certain eels might be of value in treating mental disease, he administered the world's first electric shock therapy. The emperor had migraine headaches, and Largus applied his eels to either side of the magistrate's skull in an attempt to alleviate his pain.

These positive beginnings took an abrupt turn for the worse in 30 A.D., however, when the first two disastrous precepts concerning the cause of mental illness were reintroduced. A physician, Celsus, concluded in his book, *I De Re Medica*, that frightening the insane might scare away what he thought were bad spirits inside them. Demon possession had returned. It was Celsus who first chained the mentally ill and tortured them in the name of healing, a practice that would continue for eighteen hundred years.

In the second century A.D., Galen, the preeminent physician of his time, despite having been trained in the Greek tradition of rationalism, again attempted to invoke deity into the mental illness equation. He sought an all-encompassing purpose for life and sickness, beyond mere logic. More than detailing how illness worked, he wanted to explain why it existed at all. Harkening back to the Hebrew formulation, Galen concluded that God and Divine Will provided the ultimate explanations. They were the unifying forces of nature.

Thus, the stage was set for sickness, mental illness included, to become, once again, a religious problem.

Soon thereafter, devastating epidemics of bubonic plague swept through the Roman empire. The populous was terrified. They abandoned rational science, which had no useful explanation for these calamities, instead turning to Galen and his ecclesiastical construct. By the fourth century, Christian dogma was being used to explain the Universe, including health and illness. Wellness was equated with piety, sickness with sin.

Priests, not physicians, began giving medical advice and performing ritualistic healings. For the brain diseased, their abnormal behavior was an obvious sign of wrong doing; grisly exorcisms and beatings became the treatment.

With the fall of Rome, the Middle Ages descended upon Europe. For the next thousand years, multitudes of mentally ill men, women and children were battered, starved, vilified and abused, then left to beg and wander the countryside to be ravaged, at will, by the masses.

Although Western civilization was in decline during this time, things were not medieval everywhere. Beginning in the fourth century, after the Roman capital (along with the ancient Greek manuscripts) was moved by the Emperor Constantine to Byzantium, the Hellenic concept of rationalism took hold in the Arab countries. Their physicians kept the intellectual flame alive and treated the mentally ill with dignity.

During this period, Arabic nations built the first hospitals which, reverting back to the Egyptian idea, contained units specifically designed for treatment of the mentally ill. Called "moristans," these facilities were created to resemble Paradise, complete with perfumed baths, music and conjugal visits from spouses.

While generally regarded as only preserving Greek traditions, Arabic doctors did make some intellectual progress themselves. In the sixth century, Aetius of Amida attributed certain mental processes to specific areas of the brain. We have only recently rediscovered this concept. We call it "functional localization," something I'll explain later.

Around the year 1000, the physician Avicenna penned *The Canon of Medicine*, which attempted to summarize all extant medical knowledge. Based on the natural principles of Hippocrates and Aristotelian empiricism, the *Canon* was the world's most important medical text for the next 500 years.

By 1100, Europe gradually began to emerge from its torpor. Under papal order, priests and monks were no longer allowed to perform healings thus ensuring the return of a lay medical profession. The first medical school was established at Salerno, Italy, and over the next three hundred years, rationalism and logic slowly returned to Continental life. Science was advancing, and as a result, lifestyles improved in many social classes.

By the fourteenth century, conditions began to change for the mentally ill as well. After ten centuries of abuse, torture and neglect, their lives got worse.

Between 1347 and 1350, one-third of the European population died from another massive epidemic of bubonic plague, now known as The Black Death. With, again, no scientific explanation for this disaster, paranoia and terror prevailed. A scapegoat had to be found.

The mentally ill, people concluded, had brought this devastation upon the populous. It was divine retribution for the mentally sick having consorted with the Devil, bizarre actions being irrefutable evidence of satanic collusion. For the next 130 years, the brain diseased were hunted down, tortured and often killed.

In 1483, in an effort to halt this nightmare, Pope Innocent VIII commissioned two Cologne University professors, Johann Sprenger and Heinrich Kraemer, to investigate the true cause of mental illness and propose any possible solutions.

After four years of study, their work was complete.

Sprenger and Kraemer's findings were published as the infamous *Malleus Maleficarum*, or "Witches Hammer," the first printed guidebook for genocide.

The authors concluded that mental illness was evidence of satanic witchcraft. The mentally ill, however, were no longer thought to be merely possessed by malevolent forces, they were themselves evil incarnate. The majority of these nefarious beings were women whose "lusts" were responsible for their condition.

Malleus attempted to prove the existence of witches, detailed mechanisms to detect them and, lastly, outlined what to do with them. The best treatment, Kraemer and Sprenger reported, was burning the inflicted alive while tied to a stake of wood. The Pope accepted these findings and a Church-sanctioned, murderous frenzy, the Inquisition, was unleashed.

Despite great intellectual strides in other areas, society, for the next two hundred years, slaughtered the mentally ill wholesale. During the Renaissance, the age of Da Vinci, Copernicus and Vesalius, the killings actually accelerated.

The era did produce one ray of light, however—the world's first psychiatrist, Johann Weyer. Studying medicine under Cornelius von Nettesheim, who'd previously written a pamphlet entitled "On the Nobility and Pre-eminence of the Feminine Sex," Weyer took pity on the mentally ill who'd been accused of witchcraft and began to study their symptoms more carefully. In 1563, he published *De Praestigiglis Daemonicum* (*The Description of Demons*), a step-by-step rebuttal of Sprenger and Kraemer's horrific *Malleus* and its murderous conclusions. Weyer's words are still relevant:

> "Almost all theologians are silent regarding this godlessness. Doctors tolerate it. Jurists treat it while still under the influence of old prejudice... Those illnesses...come from natural causes."

Not bad for 1563.

On the other hand, as it had with Plato and Aristotle, another ideological battle erupted during this time that bedevils psychiatry to this day.

Philosopher Renee Descartes proposed that man possessed a "thinking substance," the soul, which was separate from and did not interact with the body. This reinforced the notion that your body could be sound but your soul sick, a precursor to the psychological causation theories of mental illness in the 1950s.

Descartes' ideas conflicted with the views of contemporary phi-losopher Baruch Spinoza, who wrote that the mind and body are in-separable and therefore identical. This was a reiteration of Hippocrates' contention that the basis for mental disease was or-ganic. The brain was sick.

A rehash of these arguments would be central to the post-World War II debate concerning the cause and treatment of mental illness that would culminate in the 1960s with deinstitutionalization and the eventual creation of our homeless mentally ill.

By 1650, the general lot of the mentally ill gradually started to im-prove. Witch burning died down, and the status of those with brain disease was elevated from malignant demon to that of the pauper, fool, cripple, prostitute, homosexual or criminal. This made them eli-gible for the social benefits of the day. They were stored in work-houses or prisons.

In addition, special buildings began to be constructed for hous-ing the brain diseased. In Paris, the *Bicetre*, for men, and the *Salpetriere* for women, were erected. In London, Bethlehem Hospital (where we derive the term "bedlam") was built. Instead of murdering the mentally ill, they were now put away, usually chained to the walls. Ad-mission was charged for public viewing.

Beating, whipping, starvation and abuse were still considered the appropriate form of therapy. Even England's King George III, af-flicted with an episode of psychosis, was hospitalized and tortured as part of his treatment.

By the end of the seventeenth century, it became apparent that something else needed to be done. Thankfully, a doctor in Paris and an English tea merchant came up with a better solution.

Dr. Phillipe Pinel was head of the *Bicetre* and *Salpetriere* in Paris. Based on his conviction that mental illness was an organic problem, and that current treatments were barbarous, Pinel unchained the brain diseased. He stopped the indignities masquerading as therapy and replaced them with decent care: warm baths, friendly talk, music and meaningful work. This has been called psychiatry's first great revolution.

Pinel's methods were copied in England by William Tuke, the tea merchant, who founded the York Retreat. Tuke instituted, in his own words, "a milder and more appropriate system of care," based upon "benevolence, comfort and sympathy."

This movement, known as "moral treatment," also affected American psychiatry. Benjamin Rush, the so-called "Father of American Psychiatry," used its principles to found the Pennsylvania Hospital in Philadelphia.

Although really just a return to ancient Egyptian, Greek and Arabic practices, moral treatment was a tremendous leap forward for the mentally ill of Europe and America. To be sure, they still suffered from their brain disease—the production of effective medication was nearly two hundred years distant—but they no longer suffered persecution by others.

Unfortunately, moral treatment was still the exception in America, not the rule. Pennsylvania Hospital aside, the burden for care of the mentally ill in Colonial times fell primarily on the shoulders of the sick person's relatives and local community. In a harbinger of things to come, it rapidly became apparent that this arrangement didn't work well.

Families of the mentally ill eventually turned their ailing relatives out into the street because of their uncontrollable and often times assaultive behavior. In response, community almshouses were constructed, but they quickly became only squalid repositories. Many ill people were imprisoned.

For over one hundred years, that's how the brain diseased were managed. In 1841, however, Dorthea Dix, school teacher and daughter of a Massachusetts minister, was asked to lead a prayer service for women at the East Cambridge jail near Boston. What she observed appalled her. The course of American psychiatry was about to change.

Dix discovered that a large proportion of the jails' "inmates" had committed no crime; they were mentally ill. These women lived in rank conditions. Filth, disease and depravity were rampant.

Dix was outraged and set about remedying the situation. Despite difficulties at every turn, she, through a life-long effort of untiring legislative lobbying and public educational endeavors, convinced thirty-two states to build hospitals for the mentally ill. They were asylums in the most noble sense of the word where decent conditions prevailed. A true hero, Dix removed the American brain diseased from the streets, poorhouses and prisons to which they'd been consigned, giving them safety, care and respite instead.

The asylums were actually too successful. For the next century, the seriously brain diseased didn't roam the streets. They weren't incarcerated, thrown into almshouses or tortured. They weren't seen much at all, in fact, and were eventually forgotten.

This was the ground in which the seeds of our current dilemma were sewn. While the chronically mentally ill were cared for in distant hospitals, they drifted from the mainstream consciousness. As they did, old ideas about the cause of their illnesses reemerged.

It wouldn't be until the mid-twentieth century, after two global wars and a depression, that the brain diseased would again merit national attention. History's lessons neglected, the powers-that-be decided once more that the community could care for these people. Upon this were the foundations of deinstitutionalization laid.

Riots and Revelations in a Tin Box

I'D LIKE TO REPORT THAT IN MY MOMENT OF INSIGHT, staring into those faces at the shelter, I wept or embraced someone in a new-found spirit of understanding, but that didn't happen. Instead, I stood in line for bedding like everyone else, found a spot on the floor and curled up tightly, trying to believe it was all only a dream, an ugly nightmare. Nearby, an electrical transformer exploded, the bang reverberating through the shelter like a sonic boom. Wincing, I thought about Linda and the boys. Would we ever see each other again? I buried my head in the ragged pillow and silently prayed. There were a string of similar explosions over the next few hours, each one making me cringe as hard as the first.

Sometime during the artillery-like barrage, I noticed a young man lying diagonally across from me. He obviously had AIDS. Shockingly thin, he had swollen lymph nodes the size of golf balls in his neck. The purple blotches of Kaposi's sarcoma spotted his face. Wheezing audibly, no doubt from pneumonia, he was also talking to himself and occasionally gesturing in the air.

While not a classical mental illness, AIDS destroys not only the immune system but the brain as well. People with AIDS (PWA) become demented in much the same way Alzheimer's patients do. In addition to losing large chunks of memory, PWA brains can generate voices, delusions and hallucinations. They can therefore behave like "regular" crazy people.

The man required immediate medical attention, but I knew that wasn't possible. I did, however, promise myself that if I got out of there alive, I would send an ambulance in the morning.

Gratefully, the pandemonium in the city subsided for a while, and I closed my eyes. But the respite was short-lived. Sleeping fitfully, I startled awake with every diseased hack from those in the shelter, each wailing siren or renewed transformer detonation outside.

Sometime near dawn, I was roused by a different kind of cough, one with which I was all too familiar. It was the wet rumble of fluid in the lungs, the sound of a death rattle.

My doctor's instinct taking over, I weaved around slumbering people to the cough's source, the sick young man, and pressed my hand against his neck to feel for a heartbeat. There was none. I shredded his shirt, preparing to do chest compressions. As the ragged fabric ripped away, I noticed he wore a gold medallion, a St. Christopher's medal.

Sliding the small amulet aside, I felt a sharp blade against my cheek. "That's mine," the tanned man from the night before spat into my ear. "The King gets all tribute." Blood meandered toward my shirt collar. It was more than a plastic knife this time.

"Take it, please," I said, letting the necklace drop.

The man scrambled around from behind me, jerked the gold chain off the dead man's neck then expertly went through his pockets, scrounging out a few wadded bills. All the while, his crazed eyes never left mine. When he was done, he held the steel shank of his long shiv directly in front of my face. "No tricks, or you're next," the man hissed then slithered back into the mass of sleeping bodies.

The dead man lay splayed on the floor. Instead of summoning help or notifying Big John, who'd retired to a small side room, I just stood there, unable to move or speak.

At last summoning enough courage to return to my blanket, I lay silent and still. The man with AIDS was dead, and there wasn't anything I could do about that. My own life, however, was another matter.

Finally, as the morning dawned, the shelter door opened and people began to straggle out, their feet stepping over the dead body.

A few inadvertently kicked it. One person rifled through his pockets again. At last, only the corpse and a pile of musty bedding remained on the floor.

Big John was coming toward me. "You've got a dead man in here," I said.

A pained look swept across Big John's face. "When this mess is over, I'll call the County wagon," he replied, stooping to collect some pillows.

"People die in here a lot?"

"Gotta die somewhere."

Exhaustion began to overwhelm me, numbing my mind momentarily as Big John continued, "Hey, Doc, hadn't you better check in with that answering service?"

"Jesus!" I shouted. My heart was racing. I had to get home. "You think there'll be a bus today?"

Big John shook his head. "Doubt it. But if there is, it'll be by in thirty minutes." It sounded like an eternity.

Big John stopped me on the way out. "How're you planning to ride that bus?"

I patted my pants.

"Here," he said, pulling a dollar from his wallet. "Pay me back when you can." I suddenly felt like a wealthy man, someone able to pay his way to freedom.

Before leaving, I had one last question. "You a priest or something?" I asked Big John.

"No," he said without extrapolating.

"Work for the County?"

"Nope."

"Then why do you do this?" Big John was carefully covering the young man's body with a blanket.

He stood, looking me up and down. "My sister died on the streets back in New York. Same story as most of these people. She got sick. My parents couldn't get her the treatment she needed. One day she wandered off. That's the last we saw of her. Three years later we got the call."

"I'm sorry. It was thoughtless of me."

"That's okay," Big John went on. "Everyone here's got a family that's wondering where they are, how they're doing. They all have parents suffering like mine did." He glanced at the dead body. "Another call's waiting right here."

I thought of John Doe. "Why are things like this?"

"Damned if I know," Big John replied. "But it's wrong. People shouldn't die this way."

"How do you pay the rent?" I continued.

"Owner doesn't charge us," he said. "There are good people out there. They do what they can."

"And you?"

"My folks left a little money when they passed. I make do."

Big John hoisted a stack of blankets. "Don't you have a bus to catch?"

III

Nervously standing in front of the shelter looking for the Number 14 bus, I noticed that the street was empty. Everyone from the mission had vanished. They'd slipped back into the crevices of the city, back under the bushes, down the alleys or behind the trashcans, retreating into their demented worlds of internal voices and paranoid delusions.

I gazed up. The sky was so full of smoke it still looked like night. I began to cough just as the shelter door opened and Big John walked out. "I almost forgot," he said. "You asked about a man last night. He might be a guy used to stay here occasionally, went by John Doe. Kinda nasty. Haven't seen him in a couple of weeks, though. He stayed over at the Paradise Villa. Three blocks down on the left," he added, pointing. As Big John went back inside, the Number 14 bus began rounding the corner.

Closing my eyes and taking a breath, the bus shuddered to a stop before me. The doors slid open as I exhaled. Looking up, I saw the same driver from the day before behind the wheel. With a wave, I motioned him away.

"Can't promise to be back," he warned, glancing around anxiously. Incredibly, I motioned him away a second time, and with me watching in disbelief, the bus disappeared down the street. I couldn't explain what I was doing. My journey had taken on a life of its own.

Despite the smoke and sirens, I began walking toward the Paradise Villa, a ramshackle three-story building with peeling paint inside and out. I'd been there yesterday, but the clerk had been passed out.

Looking through a glass pane in the front door, I noticed the same alcohol-withered man sitting behind a small front desk. I pulled on the handle. It was locked.

I banged on the door, but he ignored me. I banged again. The clerk peered up but didn't move. Finally, I pounded so hard the building began to shake. Angrily, the man hobbled to the door, his face framed by its small window.

"Are you crazy?" he snapped. "The whole fuckin' city's burning down. No rooms. We're closed."

"I'm not looking for a room..." I said but the clerk cut me off.

"Then fuck off."

"But..."

"Get outta here before I call the cops," the clerk growled and turned away.

"I don't give a shit about riots!" I shouted, ripping at the door handle again which brought the clerk back. "Or about cops! Or about you! I need some information, and I'm going to get it! I'm looking for the address of a man called John Doe. He's dead, and his family should know."

After a few beats of silence, the clerk unlocked the door, opening it a sliver. "I wondered what happened to that prick," he spat.

"You knew him?" I asked incredulously.

"Bastard lived out back," the clerk grumbled, closing and relocking the door.

I ran around the corner and down the adjacent alley, skidding to a stop behind the crumbling stucco structure. Before me was a sagging piano crate bruised with wear. My heart racing, I crawled through a low cloth "door" and into the cramped seven-by-four foot "house."

There were two dirty blankets on the floor with a threadbare pillow beside them. The walls were stained with rainwater, mold and, judging from the smell, urine. The rest of the room was packed with moldy trash: wadded fast food wrappers, old paper cups and wrinkled plastic bags. I saw bent coat hangers, a broken umbrella and a metal chair with no cushion. Degenerating newsprint was scattered everywhere.

Apprehensively, sliding the refuse around with my shoe, I struck something solid. Gingerly reaching down, I pulled up a rotting boot and tossed it aside. I continued searching, rummaging through pile after pile of rotting paper and God-knows what else. My skin was crawling. I jumped when something scurried through a mound of rubbish not two feet from me. Imagining a huge rat, I'd finally had enough. Card-or-no-card, I was going home.

In frustration, I kicked a final heap of garbage near the door and heard a clunk. Bending over again, I plucked a dented cigar tin from the debris. Holding it into the dim light, I examined my find. I'd seen dozens of them before. Horribly rusted but still recognizably blue in color, with a faded picture of a smiling seventeenth century cavalier on the front, it was the same type of box my friends and I had used to store baseball cards when we were kids. The container was closed tightly. Putting a finger under the lip of the lid, I carefully pried off the top and gently rifled through the contents. It was filled with a fistful of papers so wrinkled as to be unreadable. Beneath that was a set of discharge papers from County General and two unfilled Haldol prescriptions, one dated 1989. At the bottom were two half-smoked cigarettes, forty-three cents in change and a folded shard of newspaper, which I removed and delicately opened. Darkened and brittle with age, it nearly disintegrated in my fingers.

It was a section from some long-ago sports page. There was a picture of a young man with sparkling eyes fresh from a recent football tussle, posing, helmet on hip, in a triumphant stance. Behind him two cheerleaders, pompoms held high, jumped in the air.

"Stanton Leads Pirates to Victory!" the caption under the photo read. The young man in the picture was John Doe. His first name, the faded text said, was Tom. The paper came from Cedar Rapids, Iowa.

IV

Elated, I ran back to the rescue mission. In an effort to avoid another encounter with someone like the men who'd confronted me when I'd first gotten off the bus, I lingered in the shadows of a nearby alley until, to my great relief, the Number 14 bus made another pass by the shelter. As I handed the driver Big John's dollar, he noticed the cigar tin under my arm and the blood on my collar.

"Tom Stanton, from Iowa," I said, sitting down. I was the only rider. The driver nodded, checked his mirror then moved away from the curb.

As we drove through the ghetto, I stared out the window in horror. The city was consuming itself. People ran crazily into the road. Twice the driver braked abruptly to avoid flattening wild, sprinting men, arms laden with stolen goods. Fire trucks, sirens and lights blazing, pushed by us. Liquor stores, furniture stores, houses and apartments were ablaze. The air was smoldering charcoal. Yesterday, I would have said that this was Hell and its denizens. Now I knew better. This was a riot, and these were looters running through the streets. Hell was back at the Safe Haven Rescue Mission. The damned were in the sewer beneath us.

"You're a lucky man," the driver said, stopping in front of the Mill. "Just got word the whole line's shutting down."

Standing at the top of the bus steps, I shook the driver's hand. "Thanks," I said. "You saved my life."

"Find his parents, and let them know," the driver replied. "They'll appreciate it."

Bounding onto the sidewalk and waving, I dashed toward the hospital. Desperate to call home, I flung open the front door. Running across the lobby, I made straight for my office, grabbed the phone receiver off the desk and quickly punched in our home number. While rapidly rehearsing some kind of explanation, I suddenly realized that this phone was dead, too. Scooping my long-lost wallet and keys off the desk chair, I dropped the phone and ran.

I went out through the lobby and hospital doors again. There were only a few cars in the parking lot. My Toyota hopped to a start, and I was gone. Racing home, I pushed the gas pedal to the floor, skidding around corners and squealing through traffic lights.

Careening into our underground parking lot, I hurried from the car, took the steps three at a time and sped toward our unit. Birdie was nowhere in sight.

"Linda...!" I called going in the front door. Then I stopped short.

In the living room, the television showed a mob ravaging a Pic 'N Save store. Huddled together, Linda and the boys were on the couch. Their faces were wet. Linda jumped.

"You're all right," she sobbed and ran over, enfolding me. "We thought you were dead." Then she noticed my neck. "Oh my God! You're bleeding!?"

The boys dashed up and hugged me, too. "It's nothing," I said, bending down to feel their warm embrace. "Thank God, you're all safe."

After another round of hugs and tears of joy, we made our way into the kitchen. "I need a cup of coffee," I said, plopping into a chair, setting Stanton's tin container on the table beside me.

"Tell us what happened," Jake said excitedly.

"Yeah, Dad," Mike echoed. "Did you get shot by rioters?"

I was tired. "No, boys, it was nothing like that. I tried to call but all the phones are out. I got trapped Downtown."

This was a mistake. Linda froze near the coffee pot. "What were you doing Downtown?" she said coolly.

I didn't know what else to do. I had to tell the truth. "I went looking for information about John Doe. I wanted to contact his family."

"Wasn't he the guy that drowned in our spa?" Jake asked, and I nodded. Linda still hadn't moved.

"Did you get what you wanted?" she said.

"He was Tom Stanton. From Iowa."

Linda looked at me but said nothing. I knew an apology would do no good. I didn't understand what I was doing, how could she?

Linda poured my cup of coffee, flicked me a glance then walked out of the kitchen. I sat there until the coffee was cold. My head hurt.

Later that afternoon, I decided to close the circle. I dialed the operator in Iowa and asked for all the Stantons in Cedar Rapids. There were six. I got Tom's father on the third try.

"Mr. Stanton," I said. "My name is Dr. Seager from Los Angeles. I'm calling about your son Tom."

I heard the man catch his breath. "Ellen," he shouted. "They've found Tom!"

"Mr. Stanton..."

"Let my wife get on the other line," Stanton said excitedly.

Then there were two people talking at once. "Is he okay? He's been gone so long, we feared the worst. Is he taking his medication? Does he look well? It's been so hard locating that boy. He's our youngest."

"Mr. and Mrs. Stanton," I interrupted. "Tom's dead. He was buried last week. I thought you'd want to know."

"Oh, no," Mrs. Stanton said weakly.

No one spoke for a few seconds. "I have a small tin of his. And a card," I said, breaking the silence. "I'll send them if you like."

I heard Mrs. Stanton weeping as she hung up her phone. "We did everything we could for him," Mr. Stanton said. "He's gone off before. But always..." Then he momentarily broke down as well. I remained silent as he tried to regain his composure.

"We tried to get our son the best treatment," Mr. Stanton said finally. "I know we should have done more. Taken him to another clinic. Maybe one last specialist." His voice dwindled.

"You did the best you could," I said. I knew the tragic frustration felt by my patients' families. They had a hard time understanding why their sick children couldn't get help. Their sense of guilt could be overwhelming. Talking with Mr. Stanton, I shuddered inside. I knew how I felt about my boys. If one of them... I couldn't stand to think about it.

"Tom is...was...such a great kid," Mr. Stanton continued plaintively. "Everyone loved him. Then he took ill. He wouldn't take his medicine. He walked away from each place we found for him to stay. Then he'd show up at the door acting crazy and looking so awful. We tried a dozen times to keep him at home. You wouldn't believe what we've gone through." His voice wavered again. "He hit my wife with a hammer. We had to put him out. Oh, my Lord."

"I'm so sorry."

"What else were we supposed to do?"

"I don't know."

V

I slept uncomfortably that night, feeling worse in the morning than when I'd gone to bed. Sitting up, I pushed my hair back then noticed that the other side of the bed had barely been slept in. Walking down the hall, I poked my head into the boys' room. It was empty. No searching for homework. No scrambling to get dressed. Just neatness and silence. The house was never quiet in the morning. Now it was like a tomb.

I made my way toward the living room and heard the low drone of the TV. They were still running shots of burning buildings. I looked over at the door.

Linda and the boys were dressed. They all stood, suitcases at their feet. Linda looked exhausted. I knew what was coming. The familiar knot in my gut tightened two more excruciating turns.

"I'm taking the kids to my mother's for a while," she said, fishing for car keys in her purse.

"How long will you be gone?" I asked, barely able to speak the words, my heart breaking.

Linda shook her head. "I don't know. Until this rioting thing gets straightened out, until we get straightened out. Until I get straightened out."

"What about school?"

"They have schools in Arizona," Linda said, pulling out her key ring.

I knelt beside Jake. "Listen to your mother and grandmother."

Jake's hurt flashed to anger. "It's your fault," he jabbed, suddenly fighting tears. "It's that dumb job."

I stood and put a hand on Mike's shoulder. He looked away.

"Phone me," I croaked as Linda and the boys lifted their luggage and walked out the door.

"Feed the cat," Linda called back, and then they were gone. As I stood in the doorway, at least something had returned to normal. Birdie was making his first descent of the day down the nearby banister.

For the next few hours, I was in a near-comatose state. I wandered aimlessly, picking things up and setting them down, sitting then standing to wander some more. I petted the cat but even he seemed numb—not purring but lying passively, silently.

I'd never realized how big and empty the house could be. I'd always taken for granted the noise, the footsteps, the horseplay. The cooking sounds coming from the kitchen. The laughter. Seriously in need of comfort, I went into the boys' room and turned on their Nintendo. That didn't help. The familiar electronic bangs and canned music were hollow noises without the punctuation of boys' chatter.

It was a lost weekend. While LA cannibalized itself in the distance, I stared at old movies on the VCR, paced and fidgeted, but mainly, in our big, upholstered living room chair, I sat uncomfortably thinking, unable to comprehend what I'd done. Then I'd see Tom Stanton's tin box and sympathy card sitting on a nearby end table and imagine how much worse his parents were feeling. Nothing made sense.

Funerals and Barbie Dolls

BY MONDAY MORNING, LA WAS QUIET. National Guard troops occupied the city. Instead of plundering and fires, the TV showed tanks rumbling past uniformed men directing traffic with M-16 rifles.

Getting ready for work, I was a zombie. Glancing at the television, then walking into the kitchen, eating was out of the question. Two aspirin took care of my headache, but there was no panacea for my heartache. Ambling out to the car, I'd forgotten my keys. I wandered back into the house but couldn't remember why I'd returned and walked to the car again. Back in the house once more, I thought about calling in sick. But what was there to do? With a sense of dread and resignation, I found my keys on the kitchen counter and headed out.

Despite the emotional turmoil, I vividly recall my drive that morning. It's disconcerting to see an armored personnel carrier patrolling the empty parking lot of your local supermarket while the dry cleaners and liquor store next door lie in ruins.

When I got to the Mill, which had somehow stayed open during that entire frightful weekend, a huge and ominous Sherman tank was blocking my parking space. I circled under its long turret barrel, turning around to park elsewhere.

That whole week was confusion. Trying to patch the time together is like assembling a jigsaw puzzle with only half the pieces. The patient load was simply unbelievable. In addition to the usual stream of voices, destitution, drugs and lunacy, there was the extra load of people lathered into a froth by the stress of charred streets and soldiers on the sidewalks. What was normally a river, turned into a deluge. Yang, Tina, Dupree and I never worked so hard in our lives.

At home things were even worse. I missed my family so badly I physically ached. The evenings were crushingly difficult. The empty house felt like it was squeezing me from every side. I spent large amounts of time on the verandah staring into the distance, toward Arizona. What sleep I got was simply the result of complete physical exhaustion from the days' frenetic pace.

II

On Tuesday, during a small break in our hectic day, I checked the office mail. In my box was a notice for Naomi Johnson's funeral. Honored to have been included, I attended. At the service on Friday, I thought how fortunate Naomi was to have had heart trouble rather than brain disease. She got a warm, human sendoff from family and friends. There was organ music and a choir. A woman sang "Amazing Grace."

I wondered what Tom Stanton's burial had been like. What had his family and friends been doing that day? Did anyone sing? How awful for his parents not to, at least, have been able to send him off. It was the last indignity in a long string.

The First Baptist Church on Compton Avenue was packed. There were a battery of mailmen, scores of relatives and hundreds of friends. Everyone in town, it seemed, had loved Naomi. I sat in the back.

Midway through the memorial, sitting a few rows up and to the left, I spotted Jamal's mother. She was thin and pretty but with a tint of hardness in her eyes. If you looked at her face, however, you could see Jamal.

The sight of Jamal's mother wasn't what bothered me most. The man beside her, a slick black man with close-cropped hair wearing an expensive suit—he was trouble. His presence meant one of two things—drug dealer or attorney. I wasn't certain which was worse but feared the latter. A lawyer meant a custody battle.

Sadly, Jaml was bouncing like a rubber ball. Frequently raising his voice to a shout, he'd struggled with his attendant social worker throughout the brief interment ceremony. Twice the pastor had to stop speaking until Jamal settled down. He was on the brink. I tried to speak briefly with him after the burial service.

"Fuck this!" Jamal snarled as I approached. Then he kicked the fresh dirt waiting to fill his grandmother's grave. "I hated her anyway."

"That's not true, Jamal," I said, glancing at his social worker, a slim, harried Hispanic woman.

"And fuck you, too," Jamal said to me then spun and took off running, his social worker right behind. Walking toward my car, I heard the woman scream. Jamal had struck her. By the time I ran over, a crowd of adults had gathered and was shepherding Jamal away.

III

After another excruciating weekend alone, punctuated by a very welcome call from Linda and the boys, my first ER patient that next Tuesday set the tone for the following days.

Pamela C. was missing the tips of all ten fingers, had no toes nor ears, and the end of her nose was gone. It looked like she'd survived a bout with frostbite or gangrene. Neither of these had happened. She was schizophrenic.

Pamela C. was from Baltimore. One of twelve children, a relative said, she'd always been considered "slow" and a "loner." "You know, 'odd.'" With so many brothers and sisters, she'd gotten lost in the shuffle. No one knew anything was wrong until she took after her mother with a knife, stabbing the woman forty-seven times. That's when she mentioned the voices.

Pamela C. didn't go to jail. She was declared innocent by reason of insanity and committed to the Maryland State Hospital for what everyone assumed would be a long time.

Within a year, Pamela C. had been released. She'd cleared up on anti-psychotic medication and was once again considered fit for the community. Following a stint as a prostitute and three arrests for assault, she boarded a Greyhound bus to California and soon after arriving, began cutting on herself.

When Pamela C. first came to the Mill, she'd only lost the toes on one foot. Over the years, though, she'd kept on whittling. During her frequent hospital stays, many doctors had tried to have Pamela C. sent to our state hospital but to no avail. As usual, she always responded to anti-psychotic drugs, clearing up just enough to be released by the court. Back on the streets, she'd stop taking her medicine, the voices would return, and she'd begin hacking once more. After coming to LA, Pamela C. had been hospitalized forty-nine times but never for more than a couple of weeks at a stretch.

During the last year, since I'd known her, I'd taken her to several legal hearings attempting to get her stays extended. They never were. Despite her getting smaller each time we went to court, the ruling was always that the danger wasn't "imminent." She'd always promise that the mutilation wouldn't happen again, that she was feeling better and finally understood the need to take her pills. She never remained on medication; she always started cutting.

Pamela C. was homeless. She received a little money, seven hundred dollars in Social Security Insurance (SSI) issued by the federal government, but it was invariably spent the first few days of the month on cocaine.

"Please, not again," I murmured walking into the ER that morning. Pamela C. was in the holding room. She had a fresh bandage over one eye.

"Pamela's back," Bull said. "Just came over from the med ER."

"What happened to her eye?" I pinched the bridge of my nose.

"Take a look," Bull said. Ten-Trees was standing beside him grim and silent.

Unlocking the door to the holding room, the three of us went in. Pamela C. was seated at the end of a long bench near the corner. Stubby hands at her side, she was mumbling incoherently.

She let Bull remove her eye patch without complaint. As he undid the dressing, we all involuntarily stepped back.

Pamela C.'s right eye stared at us round and unwavering. She looked like something out of *Tales from the Crypt*. She'd ripped off her eyelid just below the brow.

"Think those assholes down at the court will let her go this time?" Bull remarked disgustedly, retaping the gauze swatch. Returning to the nursing station, even Ten-Trees looked shaken.

Grabbing Pamela C.'s paperwork, I ordered Haldol to be given and made arrangements for her admission to the ward. "We should have kept everything she's whacked off," Bull grumbled. "You could dump them all on the God-damned judge's desk. Maybe then he'd commit her."

After I was done, I had to take a short walk outside.

Later that afternoon, during a brief pause in the patient onslaught and with Pamela C. momentarily out of my mind, I went to sit for a minute in the doctors lounge. Yang was there, a book open in his lap. When he hadn't turned a page for five minutes, I realized he was sleeping.

Having been on call the night before, working into his twenty-ninth or thirtieth straight hour, it wasn't unusual for a resident to fall asleep during a lull. I always let them be. I'd been through two residency programs and was amazed the housestaff didn't collapse more often.

Remembering the deep exhaustion of my own training days, my mind started to drift. Through half open eyes I glanced at Yang again. Thinking perhaps the light was playing tricks on me, I stood and gently stepped closer. Yang's shirt collar was loose, his head tilted to the side. On his neck, just above the left shoulder, was a lump the size of an egg. Then I noticed that he looked thinner than usual, and his clothes were hanging somewhat loosely.

I was suddenly filled with a gnawing dread as I flashed to the man from the shelter and once again saw that dead body lying twisted on the concrete floor.

Yang startled awake. Standing, he buttoned his shirt collar. "Later, girlfriend," he said with a smile as he left the doctors lounge, not appearing to notice my silently shocked demeanor.

All through the afternoon I tried to respond to Yang normally, but found it difficult. "You okay?" he finally asked.

"I've got a lot going on right now," I replied honestly.

At 4:30, with the day shift anxious to leave and the night group waiting to take over, Bear wasn't in the ER. For ten minutes we sat and waited. He was never late.

"I hope he's all right," Tina said finally.

No sooner were the words out of her mouth than Bear walked in. It didn't seem like anything was wrong. He strode confidently.

"Sorry," he said.

During sign-out rounds, all the day's patients were handed over including Pamela C. and a new man just coming through the door. He'd been transferred from a private hospital. In medical parlance this is called a "dump." It meant the patient had run out of insurance. At the Mill, we were used to this kind of thing. I'd taken the call and made the arrangements.

"I heard him coming through the lobby," Bear said. "What's the story?"

"He's a drinker," I replied. "Got detoxed at St. Theresa's, but they say he's still disorganized. A bed should open up on the ward in the morning." Then I stood. "That's it. Good luck."

"See you tomorrow," Bear said as the day crew left.

My team had ward duty the next day. There were new patients to be seen. When Tina didn't show up for morning rounds, I headed straight for the nursing station.

"Did Tina call?" I asked Isabel, the unit clerk.

Every successful in-patient service has someone like Isabel. She knew more about running the ward than anyone, myself included. If you needed anything, you saw Isabel. If she couldn't find it, it probably didn't exist.

"Haven't seen her and no call," she said, turning away from her desktop computer.

First it was John Doe and the riots, then Naomi's death, my family leaving, Yang and now Tina. Everything seemed to be coming apart at the seams.

IV

Without a medical student, I had to do her share of the day's work as well as my own. Swimming in deep enough water, I didn't need the extra burden.

First off, I saw our new patient, the one who'd been transferred from St. Teresa's. A black man in his late sixties, his name was Thomas T. Moses. I walked into his room. He was in the bed nearest the window. "I'm Dr. Seager," I said with hand extended. "How are you?"

Moses, tall and slender, his frame bent slightly by the years, shook my hand. "Fine," he said.

"What happened that you had to come to the hospital?"

Moses looked around. "Hospital, huh?" he muttered. "Don't know. Must be sick."

A bell went off in my head. "Do you remember my name?"

Moses thought for a second. "You're Dr. Smith," he said, cautiously. "Been my doctor for years."

I'd need to do a more thorough evaluation but the man most likely had Korsakoff's psychosis, a state of permanent memory damage caused by a chronic vitamin deficiency usually due to alcoholism.

Korsakoff's psychosis, named for the nineteenth century Russian neuroanatomist, results from a prolonged insufficiency of vitamin B1, also called "thiamine." Thiamine allows your brain to break down glucose, its only source of food. Without it, your neurons starve. Korsakoff's usually follows a syndrome called Wernicke's encephalopathy, an acute situation in which a person's gait becomes disturbed, his eye muscles don't work correctly and he is delirious, i.e., seeing things and acting agitated. Wernicke's is a sign that brain thiamine levels are dangerously low and, if not immediately corrected, will continue on to Korsakoff's.

For all the damage that results, the site of pathology in this disorder is actually quite small. Two tiny structures called the "mamillary bodies," part of the brain's "limbic system" where memory is encoded, become necrotic and die.

Without the ability to remember anything, the lives of those who suffer from Korsakoff's are chaotic and unmanageable. When they can't answer a question, they frequently make up something to fill in the blanks, a behavior known as "confabulation." That's why I was "Dr. Smith."

What struck me most about Moses wasn't his diagnosis, however. It was the feeling that I knew the man. I recognized his face but couldn't place it. He hadn't been a patient of mine. Somehow, I knew him personally. At that moment, both doctor and patient were struggling to remember each other.

V

Tina returned to work the next morning saying that she hadn't been feeling well the day before. We were in the ER finishing sign-out rounds.

"I understand," I replied. "But next time call. I was worried."

"I'm sorry," Tina said. "It won't happen again."

The ER was busy. Yang, Dupree and Tina were seeing patients as fast as possible. I took calls from three private hospitals all wanting to send us people. Hanging up the phone, I turned as Bull stuck his head in the doctors lounge door.

"There's someone you should see," he commented. This always meant trouble.

Out in the nursing station, we watched as an Asian woman was wheeled into one of our observation rooms on a gurney. She had two ambulance attendants with her. A worried clutch of family members huddled inside the main door. Grabbing Tina, I followed the gurney.

"She hasn't eaten in three weeks," one of the medics told Bull as the two of them slid the woman onto our bed. Bull began taking her pulse and blood pressure.

"Name is Emma Chang," the attendant concluded, leaving some papers at the foot of the bed.

"Let's take a look at her then talk to the family," I said to Tina.

As I prepared to do a physical exam, Bull reported that Emma's vital signs were stable. She was breathing. Her eyes were open. But when I spoke to her, she didn't respond. Something was obviously wrong.

Shining a light in her eyes, the pupils got smaller. Increased pressure on the brain, usually from bleeding, makes pupils abnormally wide and unresponsive to light. When pupils are constricted down and immobile, it's generally a sign of narcotic intoxication. Emma's pupils were fine. I tapped a small hammer on her knee and elbow tendons; both reflexes worked normally. I listened to both lungs and poked around her abdomen. Nothing.

"Miss Chang," I said, shaking her again gently. Again, no reply.

Then I lifted her hand and placed it above her face. When I let go, the arm didn't move. Often people who feign illness will let their extremity fall, but it never hits them. I raised her other arm. It stayed in the air as well.

"Catatonia," I said to Tina. "Get Yang and Dupree, they'll want to see this."

Catatonia is a brain disorder that freezes you like a Barbie doll. Patients will stay in any position into which they're put. Having catatonia doesn't mean you're schizophrenic, it means your brain isn't working right, not allowing the muscles to function properly. It's not like being in a coma: you're awake but you can't move. And you're not really paralyzed either; you can hold an extremity in position but only when someone else moves it. Without correct treatment, people can remain catatonic for years.

The problem results from a drop in the action of Gamma Amino Butyric Acid (GABA), a neurotransmitter that allows muscles to relax. Administration of Valium, Ativan or similar drugs called benzodiazepines usually corrects the imbalance. If that should fail, then there is one other alternative.

"Two milligrams of Ativan IM," I said to Bull, after I'd demonstrated Emma's pathology to the housestaff. He drew up the medicine from a bottle in the nursing station cabinet and shot it into her arm. Then we waited.

After twenty minutes nothing had happened. I had Bull give the medication again. An hour later, there was still no change.

"Now what?" Tina asked.

"We'll have to zap her," Yang said.

"Sorry?" Tina looked confused.

"ECT. Electro-Convulsive Therapy," I replied. "Shock treatment."

Disillusionment, Despair and Murder

FRIDAY WAS WARD DAY. Time for some old friends to move on. There's a high turnover on the in-patient unit. Patients get better and return to their board-and-care homes, some win court hearings and end up in shelters or on the street, a number go home to their families. A fraction of our sick people get transferred to one of the County's ever shriveling supply of longer stay units, one of which is La Casa, a "step-down" facility where, for a few weeks, they continue to receive treatment while being gradually transitioned back to the community. A final group, comprising the rare few, is sent to the state hospitals. These slots are reserved for those patients we've successfully placed on conservatorship, after laboriously navigating the treacherous legal minefield. The state hospitals are a big part of our patients' problem.

In Los Angeles we have two options—Metropolitan State Hospital in Norwalk or Camarillo further up the coast. These are the kind of facilities originated by Dorthea Dix; full-service asylums built specifically for the on going care of the chronically mentally ill. They're being closed by deinstitutionalization. At "Metro," the number of beds is continually being slashed. Camarillo, geared to treat not only mentally ill adults but also developmentally disabled and sick children, is being razed. A new state college is going up in its place. Soon, we will have no place at all to put our sickest patients.

II

"Lula Butts," Yates began at rounds.

"She's improved on Depakote and Haldol," Yang said. "The board-and-care will take her back."

"She has an appointment in two weeks at Long Beach Mental Health," Salazar added. "Don't forget to write her prescriptions."

I nodded. Depakote is a new drug used to treat bipolar disorder. It's an anti-seizure medication we've borrowed from the neurologists and is beginning to replace the old stand-by, lithium, an effective but more toxic medication.

"She'll be back," Yang said, the resignation obvious in his voice.

"They all come back," Salazar replied.

"Rev. Ike," Yates continued.

I'd spoken to Rev. Ike before rounds. He was a typical example of our difficulty. He should have gone to Metro to be housed, fed and cared for in a decent manner. During his stay on the ward, however, he'd taken just enough medicine to utter the magic words.

"I'm filing a writ." It was the first coherent sentence he'd formulated in weeks.

"I think you really need to stay," I argued, but Rev. Ike would have none of it.

"There's a mission at Vermont and Century with a soup kitchen next door," he mumbled softly. "I have clothes."

Rev. Ike knew the game. I shook his hand. "God speed, my friend," I said.

"Praise Jesus and his little lamb Mary," Rev. Ike replied.

The cursing having stopped, Carlos Villegas was leaving with his family. Crystal Adams had a bed at La Casa. Colter was also going to a board-and-care home. Mr. Tran, finally assured that his penis wasn't shriveling, was scheduled to be picked up by his wife. Alexander had won his PC hearing the day before.

But there was no shortage of patients. A new crop had recently arrived: the shrinking Pamela C., the forgetful Mr. Moses, Emma

Chang, the woman who couldn't move, and others. More still were on the way.

Tina and I saw Lula before she left. She was dressed in an enormous purple and pink muumuu, which wasn't surprising; loud colors traditionally appeal to bipolar patients.

"Please be careful," I cautioned. "And take your medication."

"Sorry for the trouble I caused," Lula said. "I love you people." Then she engulfed Tina and I in a giant hug, crushing us into her pillowy bosom.

After Lula let go, I smoothed my mussed hair. "See you next time."

"Won't be no next time, Doc," Lula stated with conviction. Almost everyone who left the ward said this.

III

That night I was home alone again and hating it. I was standing out on the porch when everything finally fell into place. Linda was right. I did have to quit my job at the Mill. We had to leave LA.

I couldn't allow myself to get so wrapped up in the problems of my patients, especially the homeless mentally ill—the street crazy. What was I going to do about anything? What difference had I made with John Doe? Enough was enough. I called Arizona immediately.

Linda picked up the phone. "Honey, it's me. How are the boys?"

"They're fine," Linda said. My heart raced at the sound of her voice.

"Are they playing ball?" I was struggling to get to the point.

"Sons of yours, and you ask if they're playing baseball?" You had to admire my wife. She didn't know Stan Musial from Stan the Dancing Bear but when it came to sports, she supported the kids and me totally, at every game, always cheering the loudest.

"Pretty hot there, is it?" I fumbled.

Linda was more direct. "You didn't call to discuss the weather. What's up?"

Feeling like a nervous teenager I stammered, "I miss you all so much it hurts. LA's calm now. Have you thought about coming back?"

"You know LA's not the only problem."

"You're right," I rushed on. "I want to fix everything."

"This is something we've talked about before," Linda whispered. "We can't go through much more."

"I've decided to quit my job at the Mill," I said straight out. "We'll move. That's a promise. Won't you come home, please?"

She didn't say anything. My breath stopped. "We'll see," Linda said, finally, her voice strained. "I need some time to think."

"Of course." My elation was growing. "Take all the time you need."

"I know Little League season is coming up," Linda began.

"Screw Little League. What's important is you feeling safe and that we get back together as a family. Nothing else matters."

Linda laughed for the first time in a long while. "Screw Little League? Check the paper. Did Hell freeze over?"

"Very funny," I said. "I'm serious."

"I know."

"Call you tomorrow?"

"Sounds nice."

IV

Before losing my nerve or having the next calamity divert my attention, I decided to act on this new-found conviction.

"Got a minute?" I asked Bear the next morning after sign-out rounds. He could sense something was wrong.

"You sound troubled."

"That's right," I said. "You know how Linda feels about LA and my working at the Mill. Now with the riots..."

"You're thinking of jumping ship."

"I wouldn't..."

"You can say it," Bear persisted. "You're going to quit."

"Yes."

I didn't expect what came next. "No way," he said. "Will never happen."

I was taken aback. "I promised Linda."

"Don't care if you promised God almighty," Bear replied. "Won't fly."

"People are in and out of here all the time. Why not me?"

"It's not in your soul," Bear stated. "You'd feel too guilty. Your conscience won't allow it."

"What do you know about my conscience?"

"I've seen you work," he said. "You'll do the right thing."

I thought for a second. "You make it sound like a disease. There are more important things than this job. I'll do whatever it takes to keep my family together. Isn't that the 'right thing'?"

"You'll find a way to work things out with Linda," Bear said then touched the watch on his wrist. "Right now, I've got problems of my own. We'll talk later."

This stunned me. Bear never had problems. "Anything I can do?" I asked as he began to leave the nursing station.

"I'll take care of this one myself," he answered and kept walking.

V

Wednesday morning at ward rounds, Yang again had his shirt collar buttoned. Dupree, Yates and the rest of the staff turned when I walked into the room. Tina looked anxious.

"What's the matter?" I said.

"PC hearing for Pamela C. is this morning," Tina reported. "It'll be close. She's sounding a lot better."

"She's also a lot smaller. What time are we on?"

"Eleven."

"See you then."

At five to eleven I was back in the conference room. Tina was there. Pamela C., eye patch intact, was there. The hearing referee and patient's rights advocate were seated at the table. Mercifully, they weren't Wentzler and Atwater, the two I'd tussled with over John Doe.

The referees and advocates traveled in different groups. Once or twice a week you got a different pair. Julia Morales, a heavyset Hispanic woman, was today's referee. I didn't know her very well. The advocate, Nancy Martin, I liked a great deal. After hearings, she often stayed on the ward to talk.

Her name was actually Dr. Martin; she had a Ph.D. in sociology. Extremely bright and articulate, she'd come from a patient care background, as, she told me, did all the advocates—the position required either a nursing, social work, medical or legal degree. As well, the advocates were well schooled in the law, having had to pass a rigorous preparatory examination.

As a young woman in the seventies, Martin had worked in the prison system and had witnessed some of the abuses prevalent during that era. Particularly appalling to her were psychiatric medication experiments performed on inmates without their consent. She'd been motivated to seek redress, a common theme of the time.

Martin had viewed the mental health system as potentially dangerous and oppressive, feeling a deep compassion for those caught in its web. "I provide these people with a voice," she'd said. "Where previously there was none." But, of late, I'd noticed a small shift in Martin's attitude. She'd lost her zealot's edge. She, too, I thought, was troubled by the system. Defending the same sick people over and over seemed to be wearing on her.

The hearing went pretty much as had John Doe's but at least I felt someone was listening to me. "If Pamela C. gets released," I said. "She'll stop taking her meds. She won't attend to her patch, her eye will dry out and she'll be half blind. I'm certain the other eye is next."

"Pamela is dressed appropriately. She has a place to live," Martin said. "A shelter on Normandie. She says friends will give her money to buy food and that she'll continue to take her medication."

"No more cutting," Pamela C. added.

Morales tapped a pen on the table then leaned back. I could see she was struggling. "I believe you're sincere, Pamela," Morales said finally. "But I can't have you losing another eye. The hospital's hold is upheld."

"I promise to take my medicine," Pamela C. protested.

"I'll care for my eye and no more cutting."

"Your advocate will explain any further rights to you," Morales said, turning her attention to filling out a form in front of her.

Martin looked distressed. "You have the right to a writ of *habeas corpus*," she said. "This means if you disagree with the referee's decision, you can have a judge review your case in court." Then Martin did something unheard of. She actually tried to dissuade Pamela from proceeding any further. "But you might try listening to your doctor. He's very worried about you."

"File a writ," Pamela said without hesitation. The court date was set for day after tomorrow.

"Maybe you can help me," I said to Martin and Morales as Tina escorted Pamela C. back to her room. "You're both nice people, truly concerned about our patients' welfare. I care. The court people care. Why are we always fighting each other? Why do so many sick people end up on the streets while we bicker?"

Martin looked relieved to have been asked. "I don't like the way things are," she said. "I'm concerned about these people and want to see them treated but also protected. The best thing to come out of the LPS Act was a strong affirmation of mental patients' basic rights, no experimentation without consent, no forced ECT, access to a telephone, decent living conditions, that kind of thing. These are essential and should never change." She continued, "What I don't like is the cops being so intimately involved in the process. The patients hate it, too. I don't like the prison feel everything has."

"You know there are many more mentally ill people in jails than in hospitals," I said.

"I hate that, too."

I'd been mulling an idea over in my head. "What if the LPS and other similar states' laws were repealed? Could you live with that?"

Martin didn't think long. "Of course. The one thing I've learned over the years is that we're dealing with biological brain disorders. It took a while to sink in, but now I'm convinced. The current system was built on another premise, one that's out of touch with reality. As long as basic rights and living conditions are protected, I'd love to see something different. My cousin has schizophrenia. I think of him a lot. But this is my job. What else am I supposed to do?" She shook her head. "I feel so sorry for these people. But rights are important. Hell, I don't know," she concluded.

Morales spoke up. "I think due process is necessary—we should have a set of checks and balances—but the system needs repair. It upsets me seeing the same people at hearings time after time. Ill people shouldn't live on the street. Starting this job, I was gung-ho. Referees come from the same backgrounds as the advocates, with, perhaps, a slightly more legal slant. But we get the same training. We studied, observed, did mock hearings. We had the identical motivation—reform. I'm from the sixties. 'Power to the people' and all that bullshit." She was tapping her pen again. "I'd love to be part of something else. You got any ideas?"

I evaded that question for the moment. "What about people like Atwater and Wentzler?"

Both women raised their eyebrows. "They're in this business for the wrong reasons," Morales said. "God knows what it is."

Everyone sat for a moment. "No," I said finally.

"Pardon?" Morales looked quizzical.

"No," I reiterated. "I don't have any ideas about how to change things. But they're out there somewhere. They have to be."

"Let's hope," Morales said, standing to gather her things.

VI

At 4:30 I stopped by my office then walked through the ER on my way home. Hundley had been working that day with Dr. Patrick Evans, another attending. They both looked anxious. Evans glanced at the wall clock. "Bear's not here," he said.

We waited another fifteen minutes then I double-checked the work schedule pinned to the doctors lounge wall. Bear's next day off wasn't until Saturday.

"You go," I said to the day team. "I'm certain he's coming. I'll wait."

"Are you sure?" Evans said with thinly veiled relief.

"Yes, go." I had nothing better to do.

By 5:30 it was apparent Bear wasn't going to show.

I called his house but got no answer.

Phoning Linda to let her know I wouldn't be home that night, I'd punched in three numbers before I hung up. "I must be losing my mind," I said out loud.

The night ER staff is different from the day crew. These nurses and clerks liked sleeping late, coming to work at 3:00 P.M. and going home at 11:00 P.M. They enjoyed a slower pace. Besides Drs. Bill Larsen and Mariana Lopez, two residents from another ward team, the only person I knew well was Ten-Trees who, in nurse talk, was "pulling a double," working back-to-back shifts in exchange for time off later.

Around nine, Ten-Trees took a new patient upstairs. Upon his return, he made straight for me, guiding us away from the others.

"Bear's up on the floor," he said. "I saw him with Mr. Moses."

I looked at Ten-Trees. He shrugged his shoulders. I headed out of the ER toward the elevators. After a seemingly endless ride up six floors, I walked full speed to the ward, keys in hand and opened the door.

It was quiet and dark inside. Only the nursing station light was on. The night staff was busily attending to their new patient. They didn't see me go by.

I found Moses' room at the end of the hall. His bed was lit by moonlight streaming in through the window. I looked in the door's small glass pane and froze.

Bear was indeed inside as Moses lay sleeping. He wasn't sitting and talking or checking on some medical condition, however. Standing beside the bed, he had a pillow firmly clutched in both hands.

I burst in just as Bear pushed the pillow onto the man's face.

"Bear!" I shouted.

Bear didn't move. "This isn't your concern," he growled. "Leave me alone."

I grabbed one of his muscular arms and yanked with all my might. The pillow on Moses' face rose six inches. Then Bear swung, flipping me head over heels into the corner. Again Bear loomed over Moses.

"Stop, please!" I begged. "He's just a helpless old man."

After an agonizing silence, Bear's huge frame began to quiver as he pulled the pillow up. Standing beside Moses, he began to cry. At first quiet groans, they quickly melted into wrenching sobs.

Collapsing to his knees, the pillow still gripped in his hands, he no longer sounded human. His was the wail of a wounded animal.

I slowly got to my feet. Moving over beside Bear, I didn't know what to do. So I waited. Somehow, through it all, Moses had kept on sleeping. Now he stirred.

The frail gray man groggily shook his head, then started when he saw us. By now Bear was beginning to regain control.

Moses squinted as if he wanted to know me. Then he looked at Bear, pausing for a moment to cock his head, like someone searching the library shelf but not quite finding the right book.

Then I recognized him. Glancing at Bear and back at Moses, I saw mirror images.

"Jesus Christ," I murmured. There was obviously a long story behind this, but it would have to wait. Moses was looking tense.

"I'm Dr. Seager," I said finally. "And this is Dr. Boudreaux. Please excuse us. We were just leaving."

Bear slowly struggled to his feet, dropped the pillow, found the wall with a hand and opened the door. Behind us, Moses was propped on his elbows. "Nice to meet you both," he said, curling back under the covers.

Outside the room, I dispersed the night staff who'd gathered because of the commotion then touched my bottom lip which was burning and swollen, apparently smashed during the scuffle. Bear leaned against a wall. Wiping his face with a sleeve, he gradually pulled himself together.

"He's your father," I stated.

Bear took a second, fighting to speak. "Yes," he said. "I recognized his voice the second we passed in the ER lobby. Haven't seen him since I was a kid. In fact, he was the last thing I ever saw."

A heavy pall fell between us before Bear began again. "I was nine years old. My father was drunk. He was always drunk. He came home one night and found my mother packing. She said she'd had enough.

When he started beating her, I took my little sister up to our room. We'd watched my father hit my mother so many times." He took a deep breath and straightened up.

"Grabbing a baseball bat from the closet, I told my sister not to move, then locked the door and ran downstairs."

Bear's sun glasses were facing straight ahead. "I screamed for him to stop punching my mother. She was on the ground, blood running out one ear. She wasn't even moaning anymore."

"I've never been so furious in my life," Bear seethed. "I swung as hard as I could. But it didn't hurt him. He snatched the bat from my hands and raised it up like a club."

"Two days later when I woke up in the hospital, I was blind. He'd fractured my skull. Then they told me my mother was dead. The bastard had killed her. My sister went to a foster home. We didn't see each other again for four years."

Bear's jaw tightened. "My grandmother Boudreaux here in LA took me in. My father went to prison. I hoped another inmate would gut him like a pig. Then, after all these years, a chance comes to kill him, and I don't do it."

It was finally my turn to speak. "You did the right thing. You know that," I said, tentatively touching Bear on the shoulder. "Maybe," he replied pushing my hand away and slowly walking down the hall.

14 A National Disaster

"HELLO, DR. SEAGER," a voice said from behind me the next morning as I stopped by the ward.

Looking over my shoulder, it was Pamela C. She'd been showered. The nurses had washed and braided her hair. She was wearing a fresh hospital gown. With a shiny new black eye patch, she resembled a well-scrubbed buccaneer.

I felt terrible. While it was nice to see Pamela C. getting better, I knew what it meant. As always, she'd come around on her medication and was destined to win tomorrow's writ hearing. But I was going anyway. Futile as it was, I saw no other way of helping her.

At least I slept well that night. I'd contacted a physician placement service, filled out the application, stamped the envelope and put it next to my wallet for mailing in the morning. I looked at employment opportunities advertised in the back of a scientific journal and had circled three ads, all as far from LA as possible.

I also began to read a book I'd bought a few years ago—a history of the mentally ill. It was something I would return to nearly every night. That first evening I was so engrossed, I almost forgot to call Linda.

Thankfully, she was still awake, and the boys were in bed so we had some time to talk. I told her about the prospective jobs. She explained exactly the kind of house she wanted and talked about taking up horseback riding again. I gave her my predictions for the coming Little League season. We discussed the weather and her parents. We spoke about important things and nothing at all.

The next day, on the way to court, I picked up Tina at the usual spot. We drove in silence; she stared out the passenger window in deep thought.

Once at Court 95, we parked and went inside. Pamela C.'s case was called at 11:30.

I testified that, although Pamela C. appeared to be well, her history told a different story. She was persistently non-compliant with her meds outside the hospital and needed long-term treatment to quiet, perhaps, the voices forever. "If not," I said. "Blindness and probably death are in her near future."

When Pamela C.'s turn came to speak, she told Judge Cohen she was sorry, that, of course, she wanted to live and would continue to take her medication. The public defender showed that Pamela C. had twelve dollars, was dressed appropriately and knew the address of a shelter. Untiringly pleasant as ever, Judge Cohen asked a few final questions then granted her writ. She was free.

Ours had been the last case called before the court's lunch recess. Walking through the parking lot, Tina and I passed the judge, *sans* robe, exiting a side door. "Judge Cohen," I called, getting his attention. "Got a minute?"

II

Cohen stopped. "Good to see you, Dr. Seager," he said warmly. "Not on the stand for once."

"Nice to see you, too," I replied, shaking his hand. I introduced Tina.

"How can I help you?" Cohen said. "I only have forty-five minutes to eat."

"Can we join you for lunch?" I asked. "Is that allowed?"

"You paying?"

"My pleasure."

"Then it's allowed."

Cohen, Tina and I took my car to a small Denny's-style restaurant not far from the courthouse. He rode in front with me, holding the door for Tina to climb out on our arrival.

"You want to know about the court's role in the mental health system?" Cohen asked once we'd ordered our food.

I was momentarily flustered. "I hope that's not rude."

"Nonsense," Cohen said taking a sip of water. "Fire away."

"Actually the courts aren't what really interest me," I said. "It's you."

He seemed caught off guard. Arching his eyebrows, he finally smiled. "I'm a short Jewish boy from Queens, exiled to the Land of the Sun," he said, and we all laughed. He continued, "Seriously, what would you like to know?"

I shot from the hip. "How does someone get to be a judge?"

"Originally the governor appointed me. Since then I've run twice for re-election, both times unopposed."

"Is yours a job people want?"

"I do," Cohen said.

"Do you get special training to be a mental health judge?"

He shook his head. "You learn it as you go."

I recalled Cohen's gentle demeanor with John Doe, Pamela C. and all the other patients who'd appeared before him. "You care about these people, don't you?"

Cohen became serious. "Very much," he said quietly. "Professionally and personally."

"You have a relative with mental illness," I guessed.

"An uncle with schizophrenia. You wouldn't have believed the old state hospitals."

I'd seen pictures.

"I want to be certain those abuses never happen again," he added. "The law does that."

"But aren't things worse for the mentally ill now? Don't the courts contribute to their being homeless?" Despite my fondness for Cohen there were some hard questions that needed answering.

Cohen thought for a moment. "Probably," he said without elaborating.

I decided to press the issue. "Do you think sick people on the streets should be forced to take medicine?"

"I'm against coercion," Cohen said, his face becoming serious. "The hospitals need to spend more time persuading. Freedom of choice is an asset to be cherished."

"Even if that choice is starvation in the streets?"

"Persuasion, not coercion, is the answer."

Tina was listening attentively. I paused as our food arrived, but couldn't help wondering how someone without many cognitive skills could be "persuaded" to take medications for illnesses they either denied having or had no ability to understand.

"Do you mind writ hearings?" I began again. "Seeing the same people come before you over and over?"

"Not really," Cohen said, taking a forkful of chicken salad. "Due process is important. I'm an unapologetic civil libertarian. Someone needs to keep an eye on the system."

I remembered something I'd read a few nights before. "But does that necessarily have to be the courts? Doctors have been extracted from the psychiatric commitment decision process. Why not the judicial system, too? What about a group of citizens doing the job? We trust lots of important decisions to citizen groups. Isn't that what juries do? That way maybe there could be more of a forum, more cooperation, less contention, everyone could have a say in the final outcome. As it is, families, especially, are left out."

Again Cohen became thoughtful. "I've never been asked that before. It's an interesting idea."

We all ate in silence for a while. At last, I summoned the courage to pose my most important question. "If the current mental health laws were repealed, could you live with that?"

"Of course," Cohen said to my surprise. "I don't write the laws. I administer them."

"And if the state hospital were opened again. Properly, I mean?"

"No problem."

Cohen stunned me a second time with his next suggestion. "If you're interested in changing the law, call the Alliance for the Mentally Ill. They're working on that." He even provided a name and phone number.

I knew about AMI, an advocacy group of family members and friends of the chronically mentally ill, but I'd never thought of calling the organization for advice. "I'll do that," I said, jotting the number on a napkin.

Time was running short. "You let Pamela C. go," I said. "You know she'll probably die."

"She didn't meet legal hold criteria," Cohen said looking straight at me. "I carry out the law, and that's the law. Maybe you should have done a better job convincing her that she needed to stay in the hospital."

"If you only knew how hard that is," I sighed and Cohen didn't reply. Soon everyone was finished with lunch.

On the ride back we made small talk. I told Cohen about my kids. He spoke of a daughter. He asked Tina about her family and her plans.

"Thanks for your time," I said, dropping Cohen at the courthouse.

"No problem," he replied.

Driving to the hospital Tina didn't say anything at first. Then she started. "Judge Cohen's a nice man."

"I like him,"

"And he seems genuinely concerned about the mentally ill."

I agreed.

"Bottom line though," Tina said. "He did let Pamela C. go."

"Yes, he did."

"He doesn't really understand what we do, does he?" she asked.

"I don't think so." I shook my head.

Tina glanced out the side window. "Everyone I've met is compassionate," she said. "But our patients still do so badly. It's hard to reconcile."

"It sure is." I changed lanes near our freeway exit.

As we pulled into the hospital lot past a ragged man on the corner shouting at passing cars, Tina asked a final question. "How did things ever get so screwed up?"

I opened the car door. "That's a long story."

III

To answer Tina's question, you have to go back more than fifty years. With the outbreak of World War II, millions of American men were suddenly being screened for active military duty. As part of their induction process, psychological tests were administered. The results astounded everyone, as did the events that followed.

Forty percent of all conscription rejections and thirty-seven percent of all disability discharges during the war were for psychiatric reasons; over two million men, more than all the soldiers and sailors stationed in the entire Pacific theater, were lost to the services. This was an entirely unexpected phenomenon and eventually changed the national consensus about who the mentally ill really were.

Prior to the war, they were thought to be a "race apart," a constitutionally weakened group whose illness was a mixture of genetic inferiority and lascivious habits, a combination of bad seed, alcohol and masturbation. There was a definitive line: "We" were on one side, "they" were on the other.

This notion was destroyed when, from the above military data, it became apparent that a significant segment of the populace at large suffered from a variety of mental disorders and that these diseases didn't respect race, religion or class. The nation had to rethink what mental illness was and what we were going to do about it.

Attention focused on the state hospitals that, after years of virtual neglect, had fallen into disrepair. They'd become rundown storehouses for a huge collection of abandoned individuals, their living conditions moribund and monotonous. At the peak in 1955, there were 580,000 people in such facilities.

The first call for change occurred in 1949 when Albert Deutsch, one of two thousand conscientious objectors sent to work on mental wards during the war, wrote *Shame of the States*, an expose detailing the "horrors" in many of these institutions. Other similar media reports followed. Everyone soon concluded that the situation had to change.

But, as would be the case many times during this era, the facts weren't examined closely enough. Ironically, most patients living permanently in state facilities weren't the chronically mentally ill. The latter group—schizophrenics, people with bipolar disorder and major depression—were being admitted, treated and regularly discharged back to the community. The shame was how dreadfully we were treating the hospitals' other patients—the senile elderly and those with incurable, degenerative neurologic disorders—who'd been taken in by the state when local cities refused to care for them. Unfortunately, everyone got lumped into one big, ugly jumble.

Nevertheless, a consensus formed, and action had to be taken. Our best minds and millions of dollars were assigned to the problem. Disaster was the result.

In 1956, President Eisenhower commissioned a federal blue ribbon panel to investigate and report on state hospital conditions. Their conclusions, released in 1961 as "Action for Mental Health," led to a new national mental health treatment approach known as the "Community Mental Health Centers Movement" or "deinstitutionalization."

This policy statement was based on an apparently sound premise, Freud's psychological causation theory, which stated that a person's internal conflicts, abetted by a bad living environment, produced mental illness. By alleviating social ills and intervening early when symptoms first erupted, the conflicts, and hence the diseases, could be prevented or, at least, their deleterious effects seriously diminished. As well, the panel concluded, care for the chronically mentally ill could be more easily, cheaply and humanely provided by the local municipalities. The principles of "community psychiatry" soon gained wide government and popular support.

In 1963, President Kennedy delivered a special message to Congress concerning mental illness. He condemned the "cold custodialism" of the state hospitals and called for a "bold, new" program of comprehensive community care. He stated that, "through the application of medical knowledge and social insight," all but a small portion of the mentally ill could achieve "a wholesome and constructive social environment."

Later that year, responding to Kennedy's call, Congress passed, and the president signed, the Community Mental Health Centers Act (CMHCA) which officially shifted treatment of the chronically mentally ill from state hospitals to new "community mental health centers."

Initially, the plan worked but for unexpected reasons. In 1965, President Johnson signed the Medicare bill which, for the first time, gave medical insurance coverage to the nation's elderly regardless of income. In a single stroke of Johnson's pen, the state hospitals were relieved of their senile patients who were now able to pay for care in nursing homes.

The following year, Medicaid passed into law. This provided federal funds to state-run health programs for the indigent with no limitations on age. This further unburdened state hospitals of the young neurologically disordered. They were either transferred to other hospitals or nursing facilities more suited to their needs.

In three short years, state hospital populations had dropped by fifty percent nationwide. When construction was completed on the new community mental health centers, the numbers dropped even further. Many chronically mentally ill patients were sent home and told to visit these comprehensive clinics for their outpatient treatment. By 1968, the number of outpatient visits to community mental health centers hit 1,778,590, which looked encouraging.

So, what went wrong with the deinstitutionalization movement? Why do we have brain diseased people living on our streets? Why couldn't community centers treat the chronically mentally ill? And, as importantly, why, despite bad results, does the community psychiatry movement grind on? Some of the reasons should have been clear from the beginning; others didn't become apparent for years.

To start with, the new outpatient facilities didn't supplant the state hospitals in caring for the chronically mentally ill. They had merely acquired a new clientele, people already in the community who suffered from anxiety disorders, mild depression, substance addictions and personality difficulties, in other words, the "neuroses," problems previously unaddressed by public services. The increase in visits to community mental health centers hadn't been fueled by deinstitutionalization. Service expansion, federal money and new patient recruitment were responsible. This wasn't social policy. It was good business.

Despite apparently adequate planning, the community mental health centers simply weren't equipped to handle the staggering needs of the seriously brain diseased. Their chaotic behavior proved difficult to manage and expensive to deal with. These patients were highly mobile and too disorganized to keep appointments; they routinely refused to take medications. The clinic staffs had trouble finding these sick people and couldn't manage them when they did.

More serious than the lack of clinic support, was the issue of precipitously discharging state hospital patients back home. Everyone had assumed that families would want their persistently psychotic and sometimes violent relatives to return. These same families were the people, after all, who'd sent the patients to institutions in the first place. And, unfortunately, there simply weren't that many locatable families anyway.

Figures from 1960 show that forty-eight percent of the institutionalized mentally ill were unmarried adults, twelve percent were widowed and thirteen percent divorced. Thus, seventy-three percent of the patients about to be deinstitutionalized had no one, save elderly parents perhaps, waiting for them. For these people, there was no "community" in the community.

There was, however, an even larger problem. Despite the tremendous amount of preparation and use of the best current cumulative political, medical and legal expertise, almost every theoretical foundation upon which the Community Mental Health Centers movement was built turned out to be false. Astonishingly enough, early intervention, better living environment and local involvement, the cornerstones of community psychiatry, didn't help the mentally ill simply because internal conflicts and social conditions are not the causes of brain disease.

Mental illnesses proved to be, as Hippocrates had stated, biological after all. They occur at a constant rate, regardless of what anyone does, e.g., the persistent one percent incidence of schizophrenia. Mental disorders simply aren't preventable, at least not by any current means. It took modern scanning techniques, along with better genetic and statistical information to arrive at that conclusion, but there's no debate about this point anymore.

An additional problem, foreseen by no one, was the courts' involvement in deinstitutionalization. Fueled by activist attorneys, their teeth cut on the contentious civil rights movement, suits were filed, and case law rapidly evolved that maximized a mentally ill person's civil rights but practically guaranteed his agonizing existence on the streets. Involuntary commitment proceedings became convoluted mazes through which everyone eventually tired of maneuvering. Treatment could be refused. And everything was to be exhaustively and repetitively reviewed using rigorous legal standards as a guidebook.

As well, when court decisions were rendered that attempted to improve conditions in state hospitals, these only contributed further to the problem. When judges ordered strict staff-to-patient ratios, rather than hire more staff, the hospitals (in a move anticipated by anti-psychiatry lawyers) simply decreased the number of patients by discharging them.

The final mistake, however, was forgetting one of history's basic lessons. The untreated seriously mentally ill have never been tolerated in the community. Their bizarre, unpredictable behavior eventually drives everyone crazy. People simply don't want psychotic individuals wandering around local schoolyards, neighborhood businesses or their front lawns. In retrospect, that the severely brain-diseased were quickly marginalized to the poorest parts of town and eventually to the streets or prison shouldn't have surprised anyone.

IV

In an effort to occupy some time, I took in a Dodger game that night. I purposely bought tickets on the other side of the stadium from where we'd sat with Carlos, Lula and the ward gang. The evening was smooth and airy. The game was ugly. Losing six to one in the fifth inning, the Dodgers were in shambles. Distracted from the home team's ineptitude on the field, I began aimlessly scanning the crowd.

It was the strangest sense of *deja vu*. I knew the woman but couldn't place her. She was sitting in the next section over, about ten rows up. Apparently troubled by the Dodger's play as well, she was idly flipping through a program. I stared until it registered. It was Ms. Perkins, the public defender from court 95. The conversation with Judge Cohen fresh in my mind, I decided to venture over.

There were empty seats beside her. "Ms. Perkins?" I said.

She looked up. It took a few seconds for her to place me as well. "Dr. Seager," she said finally.

"I hate to bother you," I began. "But could we speak for a moment? I have some questions I'd like to ask."

Perkins stood. "Let's have a Coke. Anything to get away from these knuckleheads," she said, waving dismissively toward the field.

We found a concession stand behind the bleachers then, drinks in hand, began walking.

In contrast to her abrupt courtroom manner, Perkins was genial and pleasant. As had Cohen, she knew what I was doing. "Why do I do what I do?" she asked.

"Yes, I'm curious."

"There are four hundred attorneys in the public defender's office. Mainly, they do criminal matters," Perkins said. "But ten are assigned to the mental health court. I was sent there."

"Do you get special training in mental health issues?"

"No."

We both sipped from our sodas. "Why do you push so hard to get patients released?" I asked bluntly.

"It's what the patients say they want," Perkins replied, apparently taking no offense. "That's my job. An attorney represents the wishes of her client, which sometimes may not be in the client's best interests. Not being a physician, I'm not qualified to judge what's best for these people. That's your task. I don't see the doctors' or hospitals' side. My focus is narrow: Do they meet legal hold criteria or not?"

A cheer resounded from inside the stadium, but it was short lived. We kept walking. "Do you like the current mental health system?" I asked. "Doesn't it seem that a lot of sick people get released?"

Perkins thought for a moment. "It's probably not that many. But, again, I don't see the entire picture. Who knows what happens at PC hearings? Or how many *a priori* decisions are made by cops and doctors not to admit patients in the first place because of the courts? I'm sure it has some cascade effect."

I asked Perkins the same question I'd asked Cohen. "Do the courts contribute to the homeless mentally ill?"

She took a different tack. "The problem is the community. There's a void. An absolute lack of involvement. If more outpatient services were available, things would be different."

I continued on. "Do you like the LPS?"

On this Perkins was firm. "The safeguards are paramount. When a detained person voices a protest, there's a mechanism to be heard. That's important."

"I agree," I said, then thought of Pamela C. "But does it have to be adversarial? Why can't we be more cooperative?"

Perkins stopped. "You know, that's always bothered me too. I understand it's difficult to testify against your own patient. And I hate the fact that families are left out. It must be agonizing for parents to see their children in such terrible shape. They must feel so helpless."

I cut to the chase. "Could you live with another type of system? Perhaps based on a medical model rather than a legal one?"

"Of course," Perkins said. "But it would have to have internal checks. There must be a basic form of review that will withstand any change in public opinion. We can never return to the abuses of the past."

"The abuses of the present seem worse than those of the past." I interjected.

Perkins thought for a moment. "Interesting point. You may be right. But whatever system we build, it has to weather the vicissitudes of society. We can never put people away again and forget about them."

"No one wants that," I concurred.

"Maybe you don't. And maybe not now. But who knows what direction the future will take. What if the economy changes? What if doctors change? I care for these people. Freedom is important. Due process is important."

I nodded. "If an administrative balance was built in, you'd be satisfied?"

"Probably," Perkins said. "Changing the law is quite a project. You'll need to educate the public. The average person doesn't have the faintest idea what you and I do. There's not much understanding about the legal system or about mental illness in general."

"That shouldn't be confused with people not caring," I said remembering Big John. "And I'm not sure about changing anything. Right now I'm mainly confused."

Perkins smiled. "Aren't we all," she said. Then the crowd roared again. "I'd better go. Maybe those fools have finally done something good."

Perkins walked a few feet then turned back. "You know you've got a snowball's chance in hell of doing anything about any of this." A bit of the courtroom bulldog flashed across her face.

Hope and Quiet Desperation

AFTER ER SIGN-OUT ROUNDS THE NEXT MORNING, Tina and I stopped by the ward to check on Emma Chang. She'd been there for two days and still hadn't moved. We were reaching a critical point. Emma was getting intravenous fluid but only a minimum of calories. She was receiving Ativan injections every six hours but to no avail. Yang had ordered a CAT scan of her head, a battery of blood tests, an electrocardiogram (EKG) and urine tests, the results of which were all normal. It's standard medical practice in cases like Emma's in which consciousness is altered, despite being fairly clear on the diagnosis, to check for other problems as well. A CAT scan is a fancy X-ray that gives a look at the brain *in toto*. It shows tumors, evidence of strokes or other gross structural abnormalities. The EKG assured us that her heart was beating properly, and the urine samples scanned for drug use or kidney problems. The blood work included a complete blood count, search for anemia, or infection, a blood sugar level and levels of electrolytes (the basic chemicals in your blood, e.g., sodium, potassium and chloride), as well as some general screens of pancreas and liver functions.

"Emma," I said shaking her arm. She was in a double room with Mavis Lincoln, a woman suffering from bipolar disorder.

"She don't say nuthin'," Mavis called through the curtain that separated their beds. "Most boring roommate I ever had. Ain't never bad." Then she broke out in loud peals of laughter. "Ever had, never bad," she howled. Mavis was "clanging," the stringing together of random words with similar sounds. This is either avant-garde poetry or, more generally, a symptom of psychosis.

Emma didn't move. "We'd better put in an NG tube," I said to Tina. An "NG," or naso-gastric, tube would be used to feed Emma until she woke from her stupor. Tina went to retrieve the device, a three-foot length of thin, hollow plastic tubing, which she then threaded into Emma's right nostril, sliding it on down her throat and through the esophagus until the tip was in her stomach. While Tina pushed air into the end of the tube with a syringe, I listened to Emma's abdomen with a stethoscope that I'd gotten from the nursing station. I heard gurgling which meant the tube was placed correctly. Emma didn't protest or rouse during the entire procedure.

I ordered liquid meals to be fed down Emma's tube then called Drs. Max Winslow and Barbara Goldberg, two other staff psychiatrists. I asked if they would evaluate Emma for ECT. We didn't take the procedure lightly. Three doctors had to agree it was warranted. Hanging up the phone, I saw a note pinned to the wall near the phone. It was a message for me to call Emma's parents. I stuck it in my pocket as Tina and I headed off the ward.

"Can I watch the ECT?" Tina asked.

"Of course." We were riding down the elevator.

"Isn't it pretty gruesome?" she said with a shiver.

The doors slid open. "You watch too many movies. It's necessary. If Emma doesn't wake up soon she'll be in serious trouble."

It was one of those rare quiet mornings in the ER. With only two patients left from the night before—both of whom were sleeping—and nobody new waiting to be seen, Bull and Ten-Trees were reading magazines at the nursing station counter. Yang and Dupree had gone to a meeting. Bear was still in the doctors lounge, seated in a chair near the corner. He had a Braille paperback in his lap, his fingers deftly moving across the pages. Tina and I sat down.

"You'll be done here in a few weeks," I said to her. "Where do you go next?"

Students generally spend their third and fourth years of medical school rotating between the various hospital services, e.g., psychiatry, surgery, general medicine, etc. This exposes them to the different specialties, one of which they will soon have to select as a career.

"I'll be on surgery," Tina said.

"That should make your family happy," Bear added without looking up.

Tina didn't reply. I continued, "How do you feel about your time with us? Is there anything we could've done differently?" Bear's head didn't move but his fingers stopped.

Tina thought for a second. "I feel ashamed," she said finally. "When I came here I knew so little about psychiatry, about the mentally ill. I had no idea how much suffering we tolerate. I had no idea, I... We..." She was battling to put words to her emotions.

"I understand," I said. "It's almost better not knowing."

Bear folded his book. "But you do know," he said. "We all know about the mass graves, the starvation, the disease. The rape. The murder. Yet, what do we do?"

I stared blankly.

"What can we do?" Tina said. "People care. I care. I just don't know what to do about it. The government should do something."

"The government?" Bear continued. "Crazy people don't vote. They're not a constituency. What politician is going to champion their cause? They're invisible. If they all evaporated tomorrow, who'd give a shit? I read in *Newsweek* about a city councilman from Florida who recommended poisoning all public garbage to keep away the 'vermin.' And he didn't mean rats. Those are the same dumpsters from which the courts allow our patients to eat.

"You have to understand," Bear went on. "The mental health system itself is wrong. The idea of being sick and homeless isn't tolerable. No amount of money, studies or adjusting the scheme is going to change that. Our discussing how to improve the lives of the homeless mentally ill would be like people in 1850 discussing how to better the living conditions of slaves in the South. This is absurd when the institution of slavery was wrong to begin with, just like the idea of sick people being homeless is wrong. We don't need to fix the system, we need to scrap it and start over again.

"Slavery and chronic mental illness are both forms of bondage," Bear continued. "But we got the solutions confused. One needs freedom, the other treatment."

Tina ran both hands back over her hair. "It's too much to think about," she sighed. "I guess there's no solution. My head's starting to hurt."

I knew how Tina felt. Trying to make sense out of this mess, my head often hurt too.

"No solution? That's not true," Bear stated, setting his book aside. "We could solve the problem of the homeless mentally if we wanted to."

Tina and I sat up. This was new. Since becoming a psychiatrist I'd only heard people complain about the dilemma.

"Originally doctors were in charge of the country's mental health system," Bear said. "*Shame of the States* resulted. We can't run things. We've proven that. And, as should be apparent," Bear leaned forward, putting his elbows on his knees. "The legal system can't run it either. With attorneys and judges at the helm, neglect and suffering have been the consequence. Even Lanterman himself, co-author of the LPS Act, recanted his original position. It was in the paper. He said the law was a mistake and should be repealed."

"If doctors and lawyers can't run the system, who else is there?" Tina asked. I could see the wheels turning in her head. Then it clicked. "Wait, we talked about this with Judge Cohen," she said, looking at me.

"You talked to Cohen?" Bear said. "Very good."

"You made me think about things," I replied.

Bear turned to Tina. "Then, as you might know, the people who should be in charge are those who should've been in control all along—the people in the community. I think that's what the framers of the Community Mental Health Centers Act had in mind all along."

"That's the citizens review panel thing, right?" Tina asked.

Bear raised his eyebrows. "Now I really am impressed."

"You're not the only one who reads," I added.

"We need a middle ground," Bear went on. "With neither the medical nor the legal system in authority. Citizen review panels would do nicely. For starters, we could get rid of those interminable court hearings. It's not that doctors mind having their commitment decisions reviewed, we've just got the wrong people doing the job, people with a different agenda."

What Bear said is true. No psychiatrist I knew cared that his choices were looked at. I think they'd even encourage it, if only the opinions rendered weren't, as they are now, so often unfathomable and calamitous.

"With citizen review panels in place, doctors could give expert witness testimony," Bear continued. "So could the legal system. Families would be consulted. But, ultimately, who stays in the hospital and for how long would be up to the panel. People are basically decent. They'd never turn sick people out into the gutter or let them eat garbage. Nor would they keep anyone against their will who didn't really need help. The courts could go back to doing what they do best: monitoring hospital conditions, ensuring that basic rights are enforced, keeping an eye on everything."

"What about medication refusal?" I asked. There had to be a way out of this court-ordered warehousing.

"Interestingly," Bear said, turning toward me. "The state of Utah has already addressed this issue. They said that being placed on an involuntary psychiatric hold is *prima facie* evidence of incompetence and, as such, medication refusal isn't allowed."

"No more Reise hearings," I said.

"That's right," Bear continued. "Someone is sick and can't take care of themselves, they get treatment until they can."

"Where would patients get this treatment?" Tina asked. "The state hospitals are nearly gone."

"This is where we have to do the right thing," Bear answered. "Again, it's a middle ground issue. We tried dealing with everyone at the state hospitals; that didn't work. We've tried servicing everyone in the community; that hasn't work either."

"We need a mix, right?" Tina said. There was a look of enthusiasm in her eyes for the first time in weeks.

"Exactly," Bear replied. "We need to rethink the role of our state hospitals. We have to realize that, for the sickest-of-the-sick, these facilities really are the best place for them. Everyone says we can't reopen the state facilities, that it's too expensive, or too this or too that. Bullshit. If we want to, we can do it."

"If reopening some state hospitals proved difficult," I interjected. "Maybe a series of smaller, local units would work. The theory's still the same—access to the patient long enough for medical and social stabilization."

"Right," Bear said. "Actually, the data has been around for a hundred years, we've just chosen to ignore it. At the end of the last century, Worchester State Hospital in Massachusetts tracked a thousand people discharged from their care. After ten years, only forty-two percent had required rehospitalization. The rest were doing well in the community. The average length of stay had been three to nine months. Remember, this was before we had anti-psychotic or any other psychiatric medication."

Bear sat back. "With the advent of deinstitutionalization, even with effective medicines, the readmission rate following an episode of psychosis is now ten percent a month. That's one hundred percent in less than a year. As you know, every incidence of psychotic decompensation, especially in schizophrenics, further worsens a patient's long-term prognosis. Community psychiatry not only dumped sick people into the street, it decreased their chances of ever getting better."

"I don't understand," Tina said after thinking for a second. "How can those numbers be right?"

"They're correct," Bear answered. "I'm not sure why, but I can guess. It takes time for an attack of psychosis to clear completely, for an injured brain to return to normal. Neurologists have always known this. They don't expect people who've had strokes or major brain trauma to leave the hospital in three days. Instead, these folks get continued treatment and rehabilitation, things the state hospitals used to provide for our patients."

"You're saying a bout of schizophrenic psychosis is like a brain injury?" I asked.

"It makes sense," Bear replied. "After each 'break' don't schizophrenics get more demented? Doesn't their function decline further? Don't they lose more IQ points? It's as if they keep getting hit on the head with a bat."

"The difference might be," I added. "That a stroke or direct brain trauma is a macro insult, something you can detect with a CAT scan or during a neurological exam, while the damage from psychosis might be more subtle, maybe at the subcellular level—equally debilitating, but you can't see anything."

"This may explain the artificial difference between psychiatry and neurology," Bear went on. "We're both dealing with the same brain. They treat the lesions you can observe; we treat the ones you can't. It's just semantics, really. Brain disease is brain disease."

Now it was Tina's turn. "Longer rehabilitation, especially initially, would also lead to better social stabilization. Before someone returned to the community there would be time to arrange for a decent place to stay, a reliable line of funding and good outpatient follow-up. No more twelve dollars and the location of a trash can."

Bear and I looked at Tina. "This from someone who wants to be a surgeon?" I said with feigned surprise.

Tina smiled, then continued. "What about medication non-compliance? Once people feel a little better, don't they stop taking their meds? You guys taught me that. Remember? Human nature?"

"That's a difficult issue," Bear said. "But the California courts have already set a precedent. Very few people, however, know about it."

"Know what?" I asked, puzzled.

"It's part of the LPS Act," Bear went on. "Under the dangerousness statute. At the end of a fourteen-day hold, if patients still pose a threat, they can be placed on a '180-day certification,' a special involuntary hold allowed for persistently potentially violent people. During those six months, if the person is discharged and fails to comply with his aftercare provisions—taking medications, keeping appointments, staying out of legal trouble—he can be rehospitalized."

"The concept is called 'outpatient commitment' or 'assisted treatment,'" I added. "It's been tried in a few places and seems to work well." This was something else I'd read about.

"All we have to do is extend this provision to being sick and homeless," Bear continued. "If you're ill and end up on the street, you get readmitted."

Bear turned to Tina. "There's no law against being homeless," he said. "There have always been hobos and skid row people who live on the street out of choice. But existing that way because you're sick?

How can someone make a choice when they're demented and psychotic? That's been a consistent problem for the courts; they take what ill people say at face value. Serious mental illness often affects a person's basic judgment, such as refusing treatment when it's clearly indicated. One-third of the homeless population is mentally ill. They need special attention."

"Why doesn't anyone try this?" Tina asked. I knew the answer.

"Who'd go to the trouble? You'd have to repeal the LPS Act and write new legislation; lawsuits would have to be filed, mental health budget cuts reversed. And getting extra money to re-open and staff a few state hospitals? Forget it."

"We bailed out the savings and loans," Tina said defiantly. "It doesn't sound that hard to me."

Bear and I didn't say anything. For a while everyone sat in silence. Then we made a little small talk; finally it was time to leave.

II

As Bear, Tina and I were leaving the ER lounge—he preparing to go home, we to begin the day's work—I spotted a man in a suit near the front door. He looked confused so I walked over.

"You Dr. Seager?" he said.

"How can I help you?"

The man reached into his jacket pocket and handed me a paper. "Consider yourself served," he said, turned on his heels and exited promptly.

Opening and reading the summons, I was ordered to appear and give psychiatric testimony at a custody hearing for Jamal Johnson in two weeks. Jamal's mother was listed as the petitioner. She was suing the County children's services. This was exactly what Naomi had dreaded.

I sighed and slid the paper into my pants pocket.

Bear was at my side. "Problem?" he asked.

"Jamal Johnson."

"Let's talk."

As I followed Bear through the lobby and into his office, it took me a moment to realize that I'd never been there before.

Bear ran a hand along the side of his desk then sat behind it. He got right to the point. "That was a subpoena, I presume?"

"Yes," I said, rubbing my forehead. "How do I always get myself into things like this? What's the matter with me?"

"You're a do-gooder. And nice guys finish last around here. The ghetto eats people like you for lunch."

"I'm beginning to understand that," I stated. "I may be dull, but I'm trainable."

"When's the hearing date?"

"Two weeks from today."

"You going to be ready?"

I looked down at the floor. "Not even close. You think you might..." I began but Bear was already shaking his head.

"I've been kicked in the teeth enough for this and the next lifetime."

"I understand," I replied. Then an impulse struck me. I was desperate. "Would you like to at least meet the kid? Maybe you can... I don't know..."

Bear paused. The pain was obvious on his face. Drumming his fingers along the desk, he put his head back. "It's against my better judgment," he said finally. "But, okay, I guess. When?"

"Two o'clock, Wednesday," I said gratefully. "I think you'll like him."

Bear face was stern. "I'm doing this for you, not him," he said.

 # Cuckoo's Nest Revisited

BEFORE LEAVING WORK, I remembered the note from Emma Chang's parents. Sitting in the ER doctor's lounge, I phoned them. We'd spoken the day of Emma's admission.

"Mr. Chang," I said. "This is Dr. Seager from the hospital."

"Thank you for calling," Chang said, the worry evident in his voice. "We saw Emma last night. She looks so sick. What can we do?"

"You're doing everything you can," I assured him. "And so are we. We have a feeding tube in place. But the medication doesn't seem to be working. We need something more."

I explained ECT to Mr. Chang. "We'd like to administer the first treatment sometime next week. Don't worry, I'll see you on the ward. We'll talk before then."

"Anything you think will help Emma, Doctor," he said.

"Do you understand what's wrong with her?" I asked.

Chang breathed audibly. "I read different things. All I know for sure is that she keeps stopping her medication and getting sick. Then she wanders off, sometimes for months at a time. We're at the end of our rope, Doctor Seager. We're not getting any younger. It's just so difficult."

"Have you heard about AMI?" I asked. "The Alliance for the Mentally Ill. They're a support group for parents with mentally ill children. Thousands of people are having serious problems, just like you and your wife. AMI has literature and information. They have regular meetings. I think they can help."

Earlier in the week I had called the number Judge Cohen had given me, and my improved understanding of this group had convinced me of the vital role it plays. AMI, formed in the early 1970s in Madison, Wisconsin, is the most effective advocacy group for the mentally ill. As parents, the members understand the grinding human toll exacted upon their ill children by the current mental health system. They lobby for bigger state budgets, better living conditions and, thankfully, are looking into changing many state commitment laws. They're currently the best hope for real change.

After speaking with Mr. Chang, with no one waiting for me at home, I hung around the hospital longer than usual. Just before sunset, I decided to take a drive and headed for the beach.

Turning off Pacific Coast Highway, then down Catalina and finally onto the Strand, I entered another world. On one side of the street were pristine sand and the dark ocean, on the other, miles of tony, three-story condominiums overlooking the water. I pulled over and parked.

It was dusk. The sun, a half crescent of deep orange, was just dropping behind the watery horizon. I began to walk, the sand warm beneath my feet. Silently passing a few stragglers heading back to their cars, my mind was in Arizona.

I was rehearsing something to say to Linda, some speech, some phrase that would make her see how serious I was about changing things, how desperately I needed her and the boys back home.

After about a quarter mile, I noticed a log washed up on shore. Passing by, however, the all-too-familiar smell struck me. It was the stench of human excrement—old human excrement.

I stopped to look. It wasn't a log on the sand after all; it was a man. He seemed to be sleeping. Around his neck, little sun-baked, molded animal charms were hung on a ragged shoelace. He had bulges in his pockets and lumps in his socks. That was where he must have kept his raw material, his clay, so to speak. He'd made the necklace pieces from his own feces.

I'd seen a few people like this during my days at County General. The man was a member of the earth's most far-gone group. He was a schizophrenic shit saver.

"Judas, Jesus, Satan," the man mumbled. He wasn't sleeping but simply staring off into the sky.

"Do you need any help??" I asked.

"Fuck off, whore!" the man shouted, his eyes never deviating from the heavens.

Sadly, I walked away. Even the beach was infected with misery. Back at the car, my radio had gone dead.

After arriving home, I called Linda.

"She and the boys packed up this morning," my mother-in-law said. "Everyone's on the road. She wanted to surprise you. We're all so glad you finally decided to get out of that terrible place," she added. I don't recall saying goodbye. My mind was suddenly going a million miles an hour.

For the next two hours, I checked the clock repeatedly to be certain it hadn't stopped. Then a familiar-sounding car pulled into the downstairs garage.

Dashing around the front of our condo, I arrived in time to see the door open at the bottom of the stairs. Jake appeared, followed by Mike, each dragging a suitcase.

The boys looked up. "Dad!" Jake shouted. Dropping his bag, he ran up the steps with Mike right behind. I knelt and pulled the boys in tight.

Then the door opened again. It was Linda. With the boys still draped around my waist, I watched her walk up the stairs.

I lifted Linda off the ground, I was so glad to see her. She was also emotional but had more on her mind than a heartfelt homecoming.

After our embrace, she took me by the elbows. "Tomorrow we start packing."

And that's what we did. For the next week, when I got home from work, we filled boxes with pictures and photos wrapped in old newspaper. We sorted books and emptied drawers. We didn't know where we were going, but we were definitely going.

Much to Linda's delight, I began receiving responses to my job inquiries. As they arrived in the mail, she read each one carefully then consulted a map. The letters were stacked on the dining room table in order of their geographical preference; one from North Carolina was on top.

Wrapped in the thrill of having my family back, I forgot to tell Linda about Jamal Johnson's court proceedings. Or, maybe, I didn't tell her because she didn't ask. My excuse was I had other things on my mind.

II

Yang phoned me at home on Sunday. He was the on-call resident. The nurses had asked him to check Emma.

"Her blood pressure's getting low," he said. "And her heart rate is down to fifty. I'm worried."

I was concerned too. Those were signs of impending cardiac failure due to chronic starvation. Emma's feeding tube wasn't enough. She had to wake up.

"Give her another dose of Ativan, have the medicine resident check her, then get back to me," I said, trying to remember the phone numbers for Winslow and Goldberg.

Luckily, I was able to locate the other two physicians who agreed that ECT was now an emergent necessity. I scheduled an operating suite for 7:30 the following morning, arranged for an anesthesiologist to be present, then called Emma's parents. They were understandably terrified. "We have to do ECT tomorrow," I said to Mr. Chang. "Time is running out."

In 1934, based on the assumption that epilepsy and schizophrenia were mutually exclusive disorders, Ladislas J. von Meduna, a psychiatrist from Budapest, began producing seizures in mentally ill patients by chemical injection, attempting to decrease their psychosis. After a convulsion, the people's mental states improved markedly.

Four years later, building on the success of Meduna's work, Ugo Cerletti and Lucio Bini, psychiatrists in Rome, (ironically the home 1,900 years before to Largus of electric eel fame) posited that seizures could more easily and safely be induced by electricity. When the procedure was administered to psychotic patients, Cerletti and Bini reported the same excellent results. It wasn't the electricity, *per se*, that made deranged people better; it was the brain spasms they induced. Thus ECT, electro-convulsive-therapy, was born.

ECT wasn't the first modern attempt at a biological cure for mental illness, nor was it the only successful one. After the turn of the century, hydrotherapy, soaking psychotic persons in alternating tubs of hot and cold water, was introduced. It decreased the death rate secondary to severe manic agitation from fifty percent to ten percent. Dr. Julius Wagner-Jauregg observed that insane patients suffering from cerebral syphilis improved after contracting malaria and experiencing bouts of high fever. In 1917, he began intravenously administering malaria-infected blood into chronically mentally ill patients to reproduce that feverous state. At the time, patients with cranial syphilis occupied a huge number of long-term psychiatric beds. Fever therapy killed the bacteria in their heads, and many were cured. For his work, Wagner-Jauregg received the Nobel Prize, the only psychiatrist ever to be so honored.

In 1927, working on the theory that insulin was a general tonic for the feeble, Manfred Sakel, a Berlin physician, administered it to persistently crazy patients, producing an "insulin coma" which made the person's mental symptoms abate. Antonio Egaz Moniz, a Portuguese neurosurgeon, perfected "frontal lobotomy" in 1937, predicated upon his idea that psychosis resulted from a bad electrical circuit in the brain and that by severing it, disordered thinking would diminish. In the 1950s, Dr. Walter Freeman of George Washington University modified the procedure. Instead of a formal operating room procedure, he performed the task by inserting an ice pick up through a patient's nose or under the eyebrow and into the brain. The process soon became so refined that a mobile "lobotomy van" traveled between the nation's state hospitals doing scores of lobotomies each week. Despite its emotionally charged name, frontal lobotomy actually helped many patients. Their psychotic symptoms often dissipated, they were less combative and, when tested, IQ scores improved. Lobotomy was so revolutionary, in fact, that Moniz also received a Nobel prize.

Prior to the advent of Thorazine, psychosis was treatable, but the measures were extreme. This, unfortunately, didn't sit well with the social tenor of the time. Lobotomy and ECT came into vogue in America, during the era of the "anti-psychiatry" movement. The psychological and social causation theory of mental illness, espoused by Freud's followers and social scientists of the day, were firmly entrenched. Supported by popular books, *The Myth of Mental Illness* by Thomas Szacz and *The Divided Self* by Ronald D. Laing, both respected psychiatrists, an opinion began to form that perhaps mental illness wasn't really an illness at all, but rather a voyage of "discovery," or merely politically intolerable, aberrant behavior. Any treatment efforts were seen not as medical interventions, but as authoritarian attempts at compulsion.

The movement reached its zenith with the theatrical release of *One Flew Over the Cuckoo's Nest*, an adaptation of author Ken Kesey's bestseller. In the film, both lobotomy and ECT are presented in a graphic and unsettling manner, punitive and draconian. This perception has persisted to this day.

While effective anti-psychotic medications alleviated the need for most of the century's other biological therapies, ECT remains. It's still the best-known remedy for psychotic depression, persistent catatonia and insanity in the medically ill or elderly. In its modern form, ECT is not the traumatic event people imagine.

Electricity is a normal bodily phenomenon, a point rarely considered when ECT is mentioned. All muscle, brain, heart and nerve cells need it to perform their respective functions. Also, other medical specialties use it routinely. Neurologists test the integrity of damaged nerves by inserting electrical probes to stimulate muscle contraction. Cardiologists and emergency room specialists regularly correct abnormal heart rhythms by shooting a surge of current through the chest. And the "E" in EKG and EEG, routine medical heart and brain tests, stands for "Electro" a derivation of "electric."

As Monday morning approached, we were preparing to put a charge of electricity to good use.

III

The ECT crew assembled early. We met in a hospital hallway just outside operating room number two, on the second floor. Dr. Goldberg, Dr. Mackey, the anesthesiologist, and I would administer the procedure. Tina, Yang, Hundley and Dupree were there to observe. We'd all changed from street clothes into surgical "scrubs," those loose fitting green shirts and tops worn so often by medical personnel.

Emma was wheeled into the operating room as we all followed. Two nurses transferred her to a stationary operating table. While Goldberg and I checked and calibrated the ECT machine, a small shoe-box sized affair which would provide the necessary electrical current, a mild sedative was administered to Emma intravenously. I placed two round patches on her head just above the left ear, to which wires were attached that ran to the ECT machine.

Thus prepared, Emma was given a dose of IV Brevital, a short-acting anesthetic which quickly put her to sleep, followed immediately by Anectine, a muscle relaxer to momentarily paralyze her. A "bite block" was placed in her mouth to prevent Emma's teeth from inadvertently clamping down on her tongue. She was given a few puffs of oxygen from a hand-held mask, and we were ready.

Everyone stood back as Goldberg flipped a switch on the side of the ECT machine. For the next thirty seconds, as the electricity was administered, Emma's body didn't move; only her big toe twitched nearly imperceptibly. Then it stopped.

"That's all?" Tina said, realizing everything was over.

"Correct," I replied, removing the electrodes from Emma's head as Goldberg oxygenated her until she was breathing on her own again.

As Emma was moved to the recovery room, where she would remain until the effects of the Brevital and her seizure had fully cleared, Goldberg, Mackey, the housestaff and I changed back into our regular clothes. Before leaving, I checked on Emma one more time. Her vital signs were stable. She was breathing. But she still wouldn't respond. Usually the therapeutic benefits of ECT take a while, so I wasn't excessively concerned. We could only wait and hope.

Yang, Dupree, Tina and I had time for a short breakfast before ward rounds. When we arrived, the rest of the staff was gathered around the conference room table.

"How'd everything go?" Yates asked. The whole group looked worried.

"Fine," I said. "We'll see."

"I hope Emma will be okay," Townes added. "Her parents are so nice."

"I hope so, too," I replied.

"Amen, girlfriend," Yang commented. For once, Yates didn't react. Instead she added, "We're all praying for her."

Rounds lasted an hour. When everyone else had left the room, Yates gently pulled me aside. She looked distressed.

"Is everything all right?" I asked.

"No," she stuttered then put a hand over her mouth as if to stifle a sob.

I knew Yates had two girls not much older than my boys. "Is it your family? Are the girls all right?"

Yates took a breath. "Yes, it's family—our family here. The night nurse overheard Dr. Yang talking on the phone to his...ah...to his..."

"Partner." I finished her sentence.

"Yes," Yates said, apparently grateful she hadn't had to utter the syllables herself. "He mentioned a lump on his neck. The nurse thought he might have been crying."

"Oh, Jesus," I moaned.

"Will you talk to him?" Yates said, practically wringing her hands. "You know what those people do. I mean, who really knows?

There are just so many diseases now. I think he might have...you know..."

"AIDS?"

Yates nodded. This was a facet I'd never seen of her. Suddenly not the efficient Head Nurse or Warrior-for-God, she was a woman and mother.

"I'll talk with him," I said sincerely. "I didn't know you cared so much for Andrew."

"We're all God's children," Yates said, regrouping.

"That's true. But Andrew's special, isn't he?"

Yates finally smiled. "Yes, he is. We may not seem to get along but... Oh, never mind. Please don't tell anyone we had this conversation."

"Of course not," I promised.

After Yates left, I found Tina and we discussed her patients in more detail. At 11:30, I went to lunch.

Walking down the hall, I saw Emma being returned to the ward from the recovery room and went over to check her. She still wasn't talking or moving, but her vital signs were steady.

On the way out, I passed Yang sitting in the nursing station. Food would have to wait. "Let's talk," I said through the open door. Without a word, he closed the chart in which he'd been writing and followed me back to the conference room.

Sitting at one end of the long table, Yang unconsciously tugged at his shirt collar. I dragged a chair around directly in front of him. "Let's see it," I said simply.

Yang knew what I meant. He unbuttoned his collar, turned his chin slightly and closed his eyes.

"May I?" I said, standing.

Yang nodded.

Tugging his shirt away from the skin, I began to examine the lump on Yang's neck. It was clearly an enlarged lymph gland. When I touched it, however, Yang didn't grimace. I ran two fingers up the back of his neck along the line of other lymph nodes I knew were there. Nothing else was swollen, which was unusual. Generally, in an infection, all the nodes in a chain become engorged. Still, I was worried. I sat down again.

"Have you been tested for HIV?"

Yang lowered his head. "I've never had that done," he said quietly.

My job wasn't to judge. "How long have you and Mark been together?" I'd met Mark at a psychiatry department social event and liked him a great deal. Although a bit older than Andrew, it was apparent they cared enormously for one another and were a stable couple.

Yang was abruptly filled with emotion. "We met my first year in medical school," he said haltingly. "He's the only person I've ever been with."

The test results now carried implications beyond Yang's physical health. "If you test positive, that might mean Mark has been unfaithful. So, if you don't get tested..."

"Something like that," Yang murmured.

Still, that one swollen lymph node bothered me. There had to be more.

"You allergic to anything?"

Yang looked confused. "Not that I know of."

"Taking any medication?"

He paused. "I'm on Tegretol. For epilepsy. It's under control. No one else knows."

"No problem," I said. I was thinking.

"You've dropped some weight."

"A new diet. Don't want to lose my girlish figure." Even in distress Yang kept his sense of humor.

"Have you had the flu or a cold recently?" I was fishing.

"I feel fine."

I looked at Yang's neck again. AIDS was the only answer. I was about to speak when, unexpectedly, some long-stored fact came to me.

"It may be the Tegretol," I said, and Yang looked at me quizzically. "I'm not certain," I cautioned. "But somewhere I remember reading that isolated lymph node enlargement is a side effect of the drug."

Yang's face was suddenly a picture of expectant hope. "Do you think?"

"It's possible. Talk to your doctor. Maybe he can switch medicines." I put my hand firmly on Yang's arm. "Get tested either way."

"I will... I don't know," he sputtered. "No, no, of course, yes." Then he put a palm to his chest. "Poor Mark. What I've put him through."

I sat with Yang for a while then glanced at my watch. I had five minutes before my meeting with Jamal Johnson. "Gotta go," I said standing.

"Thank you," Yang said sincerely.

"You're welcome," I replied and left the room.

Walking toward the elevator I thought, "Jesus, I hope I'm right."

Not Your Typical Day in Court

WHEN I GOT DOWN TO MY OFFICE, Jamal and his social worker were waiting outside. I recognized the woman from the funeral.

"Teresa Reyes," she said.

"It's a pleasure," I replied, shaking her hand.

Standing quietly, Jamal had on a white shirt with a red bow tie. I hardly recognized him. "Hi, Doc," he said, grinning.

I stepped back in bewilderment. "What happened? Jamal looks so...good."

A gleam of motherly pride passed across Reyes' face. "The doctor at the group home prescribed a new medication," she said reaching over to smooth Jamal's hair. "It's been fantastic. He's getting along with the other kids. His grades are improving." Then she took a deep breath. "That's why this is so tragic. I assume you got notice of the custody hearing? If he goes back to his mother, he'll lose all the ground he's gained."

I was about to reassure Reyes when Bear walked up. Jamal stared up at him like he was Godzilla.

"Dr. DuBerry Boudreaux," I said. "Teresa Reyes, Jamal's social worker." Reyes instantly grasped the situation, found Bear's hand and shook it. "I asked Dr. Boudreaux to stop by and meet Jamal. I hope you don't mind?"

Reyes smiled. "Of course not. We need all the help we can get."

"And, Bear," I turned slightly. "This is Jamal Johnson."

Jamal extended his hand, as did Bear, but they didn't meet.

"You blind?" Jamal asked.

"Yes," Bear said, finally locating Jamal's palm.

"Jamal..." Reyes tried to interrupt.

"How'd you get that way?" the boy continued.

"My father beat me," Bear said.

Jamal nodded. "I been beat a lot in my life, too."

For a second, the two kept a grip on each other.

"Let's go inside," I said, unlocking the door to my office. Jamal took a seat next to Bear, and we all talked for the next hour.

At the end of the session, I hoped Bear might have changed his mind about what I was trying to do. "Liking the kid only makes it hurt worse," he said after Jamal and Reyes left.

Then he walked out the door. "What the hell am I doing?" I moaned, slumping into the chair behind my desk. I looked over at Ken Stabler. He didn't have an answer.

II

The next three days began expectantly with each new ECT treatment for Emma, but by the afternoon, nothing had changed.

Her blood pressure was lingering at ninety over sixty, barely tolerable.

"What if ECT doesn't work?" Tina asked as we stood by the bedside on Thursday before going home.

"I don't want to think about that," I said.

That night I went to bed long after Linda and the boys. I tried to watch TV but mainly paced, unable to get Tina's question out of my mind.

Friday morning I stopped by the ward before heading up to the OR. "Dr. Seager," said a woman I didn't recognize. Her hair was combed. She wore a new dress.

"Yes," I uttered hesitantly.

"Doesn't she look terrific?" Yates effused, standing by her side. "It's Emma. She woke up last night. Hundley pulled out the NG tube and stopped her IV. After we helped her shower, she ate breakfast."

I walked over and took Emma's hand. "Glad to meet you," I said. "A lot of people were very worried."

"Thanks so much," Emma replied softly. She hadn't spoken in weeks.

"You won't stop taking your medication again?" I asked.

"I promise," Emma said.

Tina and Yang came through the door. "Oh, my God," Tina gasped.

"Emma!" Yang shouted. "Good to see you, girlfriend!"

"I wouldn't believe it if I hadn't seen it," Tina said.

I called Emma's parents. Her father cried on the phone.

III

That night I planned to tell Linda about Jamal Johnson's hearing. She had to know because if Bear was wrong and we won, I was prepared to become Jamal's legal custodian. Being responsible for another child was something I hadn't worked through completely. Could we move then? Even if Jamal stayed in the group home, how would I supervise his care from North Carolina? Linda needed to understand what was at stake. I needed to find the right moment to explain things.

We had dinner, packed a few boxes, then put the boys to bed. I'd rented my favorite movie, *Harvey*, with Jimmy Stewart—the one about the six-foot invisible rabbit. I put the tape in the VCR, and we settled on the couch. As I slid an arm around Linda, she nestled into my shoulder.

By 11:30 she was asleep and *Harvey* was over. I hadn't said anything about Jamal. Linda was resting so soundly beside me, I covered her with a blanket then went to bed. I tossed and turned all night.

"You still here?" Linda said the next morning. She'd already been up and out.

I roused and rubbed my eyes. "Where should I be?"

"It's Saturday, June second. Doesn't that ring a bell?" Linda walked into the bathroom.

I sat on the edge of the bed. "So?"

She popped her head back through the doorway. "Kill the umpire?"

"Holy Christ!" I shouted, leaping to my feet and grabbing a small nightstand clock. "Why'd you let me sleep so late? I'll miss the eight-year olds!" Madly scrambling for my clothes, I struggled to pull on a pair of sweat pants, hopping from one foot to the other.

"Where are the boys?" I mumbled through a shirt pulled over my head.

"They've been at the park for half an hour," Linda called out. The shower was running.

"Shit," I said, lacing my sneakers. I threw on a hat, snatched my rosters off the dresser and was out the door.

When I returned that afternoon with the player sheets only half-filled, Linda knew something was wrong.

"A lot of kids didn't show?" she asked, picking up my clipboard and flipping through the pages.

I was sitting at the kitchen table. "The kids were fine. Best turn out ever."

Linda took a seat across from me. "I probably don't want to hear it, but something's bothering you. Spit it out."

There was nothing to do but come clean. "Do you recall when I spoke about Jamal and Naomi Johnson?"

"The boy living with his grandmother who's so sick?"

"Was so sick," I said. "She passed away. Now there's going to be a custody hearing, and I promised the woman Jamal wouldn't go back to his abusive mother. Remember?"

"Is she that bad?"

"She's a crack addict. She broke his leg in three places during a beating."

Neither Linda nor I spoke for a moment. "The hearing is Monday morning," I said finally. "I have to testify. If we win, I'm asking to be Jamal's guardian. It might affect our move. It might affect a lot of things. I'm sorry."

Just then Jake and Mike came through the front door and walked into the kitchen. Their baseball uniforms were dirty and grass stained.

Oblivious to us, they headed straight for the refrigerator where each pulled out a can of soda. Their banter was jostling boy talk.

"Your team's really lame, Jake," Mike said, flipping a pop-top tab.

"Lame? No way," Jake replied. "You're the lame one. With you pitching you'll lose a hundred to nothing."

"I doubt it," Mike answered as they headed out of the kitchen and down the hall, their plastic cleats chattering softly on the tile. "Coach Dunn is going to show me a curve ball. I'll smoke 'em."

"Curve ball? You?" Jake said. "This I gotta see..." The rest of their conversation was drowned by a closed door and electronic Nintendo music.

Linda looked toward the hall, her eyes following a thin trail of dust that had only moments earlier been happy carefree children. She walked over to the kitchen window, folded her arms, leaned against the sill and stared out over the city she wanted so desperately to leave. I didn't move.

Finally, after a long silence, Linda turned, walked back and kissed me on the cheek. "Good luck," she said.

IV

I was at the Mill early Monday. I checked in on Emma who was reading in the day room. She'd gained three pounds since Friday. I rode down the elevator, grabbed Jamal's files from my office and was back on the road.

In contrast to Court 95, the downtown superior court building is an imposing granite edifice that became even more foreboding the closer I got.

Ascending the large front stairway, I passed dozens of well-dressed men and women, each with a briefcase in hand. Inside the door, however, any pretense of procedural dignity quickly dissipated.

Outside the courtroom proper, in a large tiled foyer, there were African-American mothers, Hispanic mothers, Anglo mothers and Asian mothers all, it seemed, in one huge teeming knot talking to their attorneys, social workers or boyfriends at once. The noise was deafening. Babies cried, feet shuffled, papers and children's toys dropped. Arms waved in the air. A dozen languages were spoken. Every few seconds someone shrieked.

I stood at the periphery of this bedlam, watching in awe. Somewhere in that chaos was Jamal. Bear was right. This was a hopeless situation, and any relative who stepped forward to pull a child from it would probably be granted the right to do so. I was fiddling with something I didn't understand.

"First call for family court!" a wall-mounted speaker squawked above the chaos, and everyone began filing inside. The courtroom was massive. A tall judicial bench stood in front of long rows of spectator seats, which were rapidly filling with the roiling crowd. I sat in a middle row.

"The Family Court of Los Angeles County is now in session. The Honorable Judith Stone presiding!" a uniformed bailiff said firmly as a serious-faced, black woman wearing a judicial robe entered and took her seat behind the bench.

Our case was listed far down the docket, which was good in a way. I had a chance to get a feel for the place, accustom my ears to the jargon and appreciate the manic pace of family court culture. Listening to the cases ahead of mine, I heard charges and counter-charges, accounts of beatings, abandonment and missing support checks. Women appealed for justice. Men claimed illness and unemployment. Infidelity, alcohol addiction and drug use abounded. It was like watching a bad soap opera but, tragically, everything was real.

During an ebb in the torrent, someone whispered behind me, "It's game time." I turned slightly and startled so badly I knocked Jamal's file folder on the floor. It was Bear.

"What in the hell are you doing here?" I sputtered.

"I couldn't let you get your ass kicked alone," he said. "You were there for me. I'm here for you. What's the big deal?" I didn't know what to say. Bear never failed to amaze me.

I could only smile.

"Next case, please," the judge said.

"*Cardenas versus Cardenas*," the bailiff replied in a monotone voice.

Just as a woman, apparently Cardenas number one, took her place in the witness stand, I spotted Jamal at the back of the room. Reyes was sitting beside him. On his other side sat a thin, balding man frantically scribbling notes. I guessed he was the attorney assigned to the case. He looked unprepared. Our ship was sinking.

After the Cardenas matter was settled, the judge called a recess. I got Reyes' attention, motioning for her to join me in the hallway. "Want to meet Jamal again?" I said to Bear.

He looked pained but finally said, "Sure. I guess."

It was a pleasure to see Jamal, whose face lit when Bear went over and stood beside him while everyone talked briefly.

"You Dr. Seager?" the attorney asked hurriedly, his pen flying.

Reyes stepped in. "Steve Seager, Bill Windell. He's Jamal's court appointed lawyer."

Windell nodded and kept scrawling. Then he noticed Bear. "Who are you?"

"Dr. DuBerry Boudreaux," Bear said.

"Everyone calls him Bear," I added.

Windell stopped writing for a second, eyeing Bear up and down. "I don't doubt it," he said. Then he looked at me again. "Those the boy's records?" He pointed his pen at the files underneath my arm. I passed them over.

"You want to be the boy's guardian?" Windell remarked offhandedly, returning to his paperwork.

"I promised his grandmother."

"Right," Windell said and pocketed his pen. "See you inside," he added, squeezing out a smile, then left.

"You know what's going to happen, don't you?" Reyes said turning to Bear.

His face was stoic. "You heard the confusion in there. They want people out of the system, not in it. Jamal's just another headache to them."

"Our only hope," Reyes said. "Is that his mother doesn't show. Maybe she's off on a bender..." Then she was rudely interrupted.

"Jamal! Baby!" a young, black woman said, bursting past me. She was the one I'd seen at Naomi's funeral. She began kissing Jamal on the cheek despite his best efforts to squirm away. It was, of course, Jamal's mother.

"Baby, this will all be over soon," she fluttered. "You'll come home with Momma, and things will be just fine."

"Excuse me." Reyes wedged her body between Jamal and his mother. "He's not yours yet."

The two women faced each other. "Well, he will be," Jamal's mother said. "See that guy over there?" She gestured to a man in an Italian suit wearing a flashy watch. He was the one from the funeral. "That's Leroy Burton. The best attorney you can find. And," she added with a smirk. "He's gonna fry your butt."

Jamal's mother ticked her son's chin. "Later, Baby," she said, then turned toward Bear, Reyes and me. "See you fools in court," she sneered and walked away.

The three of us were silent. Behind us Jamal was wiping his face with a shirtsleeve. "She has fresh needle tracks on her arm," Reyes said in amazement. No sooner were the words out of her mouth, however, than Burton, the attorney, pushed the cuffs of his client's blouse down around her wrists as they entered the courtroom.

"Why does she want Jamal back?" I was staring at nothing in particular.

"It means a bigger welfare check," Bear replied without emotion.

"A few more vials of crack per month," Reyes added equally flatly.

"How can she afford an attorney like that?" I asked.

Reyes and Bear both turned toward me. "She's sleeping with the guy?" Reyes suggested.

I'm a bit dense sometimes. "Right," I mumbled.

The four of us silently followed everyone back into the courtroom.

IV

"That jerk never sent a dime!" a huge white woman exclaimed from the witness stand. "Either he pays up, or I want his rear-end in jail."

For the next two hours I listened to the vulgar language and seething turmoil that was Family Court. I wondered how Judge Stone withstood all the impulsivity, raw emotion and demands. Witness after witness screamed, cried and pled. It was all finally too much. I sat back and tried to tune everything out.

"*Johnson vs. Child Services*," the bailiff suddenly announced snapping me out of my funk.

"Good luck," Bear said in a resigned tone as I stood, made my way down the row of people, out into the aisle and toward the front of the courtroom.

I sat behind a long table facing Judge Stone. Reyes and Jamal were beside me. Windell, arriving hurriedly, joined us. At another table to our right were Jamal's mother and her attorney. He had a pristine leather valise in front of him. They both looked confident.

"Arguments for the plaintiff," Judge Stone said as Burton rose and for the next ten minutes painted an eloquent picture of Jamal's mother, little of which, unfortunately, was true. He told of a struggling young woman abandoned by a savage husband then recounted in heroic detail her battle with drugs from which, he claimed, she was now clean, even producing an affidavit to prove it.

"Who issued this certificate?" Judge Stone asked. She was taking notes.

"Dr. Elias Wilson of the Crenshaw Medical Group," Burton replied with a flourish.

I had to laugh. Everyone at the Mill knew about Dr. Wilson and his medical group. They were a notorious scam outfit. You could get them to sign anything for a price. Back when they were known as the Central Avenue Medical Associates, they'd been prosecuted for selling phony narcotic prescriptions. I was certain the court knew this as well. I was wrong.

"Congratulations, Miss Johnson," Judge Stone said as the bailiff handed her the paper, and she examined it.

"Thank you, your Honor," Jamal's mother replied sweetly.

"Miss Johnson wants the return of her son to reunite themselves again as a family," Burton went on, pushing all the right buttons. "It's what she's fought for all these years. It's what she deserves," he concluded. During his entire statement, the man didn't mention Jamal's name once.

Then Judge Stone looked at Windell. "The defense."

"I'd prefer to let Jamal's doctor speak," Windell said. "If it pleases the court."

I looked at Windell. At least he'd used the boy's name.

Judge Stone asked for my name, and I gave it. Then I stood as Windell sat.

"Proceed," Judge Stone said. My spirits were at rock bottom.

"Your honor," I began and relaxed a bit. "I think the truth is different than what you've heard." I presented the facts—the history of mistreatment and abandonment. I recited the conclusions of my psychiatric report, stating that Jamal would need continued medication and close supervision. Speaking from the heart, I got to the point.

"The facts are simple. Jamal Johnson doesn't want to live with his mother. There is a documented history of neglect, abuse and drug use." I glanced over at Jamal's mother who unconsciously put both hands on the hollows of her elbows. "Jamal's in a group home now and doing well. Don't return him to a nightmare. We have reason to believe that Miss Johnson continues to use drugs. And, quite frankly," I said, knowing I was overstepping my bounds, "The Crenshaw Medical Group is a fraudulent outfit. Something very wrong is happening here. Please, your Honor, consider another option. Place Jamal under my guardianship. I'll see that he gets the care he deserves. I'm begging you, for his sake. Thank you." I sat down.

"Objection!" Burton said firmly. "That's all hearsay and potentially libelous. It should be stricken from the record."

Judge Stone thought for a moment. "Are you saying this document is a fake?" she asked, holding up the edge of the supposed drug program certificate.

I couldn't contain myself. "The woman has needle marks on her arms," I said disgustedly. "Ask her to show you."

"Objection, Your Honor!" Burton shouted, standing this time. "You have the doctors' testimonial. Miss Johnson has proven she's overcome her past problems."

Judge Stone looked at the paper and at Jamal's mother. "You don't have to show your arms, Miss Johnson," she said finally. "Objection sustained." I knew it was over.

Judge Stone took a second to gather her thoughts then showed considerable empathy in her concluding statement.

"Dr. Seager," she said looking down over her glasses. "The court is not without sympathy for your argument nor does it doubt the honesty and sincerity of its intent. However, there are certain realities to be faced here. Our directive from the State Legislature regarding family litigation is always to lean heavily toward reunification, and this court falls under the purview of that action." She continued, dropping her tense from the third person. "You spoke of other options, I simply have none. On a very basic level, there is an obvious problem here that needs mentioning. Jamal is black, you're not. While volunteering to take him under your care is commendable, it's just not practical. Besides, foster care is only temporary and now, today, permanent arrangements for the child must be made."

Judge Stone straightened up; the judicial mask was now firmly back in place. I didn't want to hear what was coming next. "Sorry, Naomi," I apologized under my breath.

"If there's no further business concerning this matter," Judge Stone stated, and I let my mind drift. I was in Hawaii, lying on a porcelain beach beneath a brilliant bright sun. Linda was beside me. The boys were splashing happily in the surf.

"It is the ruling of the court, therefore..."

"Wait," a deep voice said from the audience, and Judge Stone paused. "I'll take him."

In unison, Jamal's mother, Burton, Jamal, Reyes, Windell and I all spun around. Bear was standing in the middle of the courtroom.

"And you are?" Judge Stone asked, canting forward for a better look.

"Dr. DuBerry Boudreaux, you Honor," Bear replied clearly. "I'm an associate of Dr. Seager's and as such am familiar with the particulars of this case. It would be my pleasure to take Jamal to raise."

"Objection!" Burton exclaimed, jumping to his feet.

Judge Stone pushed her glasses up onto her forehead. "I don't know," she said hesitantly. "This is highly irregular."

Right then, for the first time in his life, Jamal Johnson took control of his own fate. He stood up. "Please, ma'am," he said glancing back at Bear. "It's what I want. I want to live with him."

Judge Stone studied Jamal's mother, then me, then Bear. The silence was intolerable. "You're blind," she said at last. "How can you handle a child?"

Bear was preparing to answer but didn't have to. "I've got good eyes," Jamal said. "I can see for both of us."

After contemplating for what seemed an eternity, Judge Stone finally broke out in a broad grin. "Then that's what you shall do," she said to Jamal.

"Bailiff, will you instruct Dr. Boudreaux where to go to initiate formal adoption proceedings? Jamal Johnson is hereby remanded back to the custody of Children's Services until such time as an adoption petition is filed." Then she banged her gavel. "Case dismissed."

"But what about my check!" Jamal's mother shouted, exploding from her chair. She looked furiously at Judge Stone then at Burton. "You said this would be a piece of cake!" she howled, shaking her finger. "You promised the money was as good as mine!"

Burton, luckily, grabbed his briefcase off the table and held it up as a shield. Fists whirling and legs kicking, Jamal's mother flew at him. "You son-of-a-bitch!" she thundered. Papers flew like confetti. It took the bailiff and three officers from the hall to drag her screaming and thrashing out of the courtroom.

"All in a day's work," Windell said after the fireworks, shaking my, Reyes' and Jamal's hand.

A joyous, tearful Reyes hugged Bear and I. "We'll get Jamal packed," she said dabbing her eyes. Jamal, however, looked strangely diffident as Bear walked up.

"You won't forget about those papers?" he asked.

Bear felt for Jamal's shoulder. "I'll file them today," he said, and Jamal finally smiled.

V

"You're a piece of work, you know that," I said to Bear as we stood outside the now empty courtroom. Reyes had taken Jamal back to the group home while we'd visited a score of offices to accumulate the appropriate adoption papers. Everyone else, with the court at noon recess, had left.

"Let me ask you what you once asked me," I continued. "Are you insane?"

Bear chuckled. "Probably. But it's your fault."

"My fault?" I said with mock hurt.

"You and all that *Leave it to Beaver* B.S. I think I'm infected."

I laughed then got serious. "That's the kindest thing I've ever seen anyone do."

Bear faced me. "I know we'll have problems—what do I know about raising kids? But I'm excited."

Bear took my arm, and we began walking. "You'll need the Little League schedule, of course," I said.

"Not that shit, no way," Bear replied, laughing.

"The games haven't actually started yet, which is good," I went on, unfazed. "You'll be a late sign-up."

"Can you do that?"

"Happens all the time."

"They still supply the uniforms?" Bear asked, as I held the front door.

"Everything but spikes and a glove." We passed through the doorway. "You might want to get Jamal his own bat. TPX is good. The boys each got one for Christmas." The glass door closed behind us.

Epilogue

I SAW TINA FIRST THING THE NEXT MORNING. "You missed a couple days of work last week," I said. "Is everything all right?"

Tina looked surprised. "I left a note." She walked over to my desk, which was covered with enough journals, mail and envelopes to start a bonfire. "Here." She pointed to a sheet of paper on top of the jumble.

I picked it up. Dated last week, it said Tina was going home for two days. "Sorry," I apologized.

"I had to talk to my family," Tina stated. "I wanted to prepare them."

"Not something bad I hope?"

"I've decided to become a psychiatrist. I thought I'd better tell everyone in person—especially my brother. He's going to call you, by the way. He's convinced I've gone crazy."

"I'm not sure you haven't," I answered, mystified. "I don't understand. What happened? Why get involved with this frustrating mess?"

"It's what Dr. Boudreaux said. There is a solution to the homeless mentally ill problem, and I'd like to be part of it. The Pamela C.s and John Does of this country deserve better than they're getting."

It took me moment to reply. "I'm very proud of you," I finally said.

II

I spoke with Emma Chang's parents when she was discharged later that week. "I called the people at AMI," Mr. Chang said. "You're right. They sound very helpful. They're sponsoring an informational series about the different brain diseases and how they're treated. There's an informal social gathering afterward. The first meeting is tomorrow night."

III

Mr. Moses, Bear's father, filed a writ of *habeas corpus* contesting his involuntary hold. At the hearing, he produced twenty dollars, the name of a shelter and got released. Bear never mentioned him again.

IV

Bear got full custody of Jamal and signed him up for Little League. His team is scheduled to play Jake's squad the last day of the season.

V

It was two weeks before Yang and I talked alone again. He was wearing his collar loose.

"I saw my neurologist," he said. "He thinks you're right. We switched medications, and the lump is going down. He was impressed that a psychiatrist made the diagnosis."

"I've had some medical training," I laughed.

"And I got tested. Negative. Mark and I are better than ever." He winked. "Thanks, girlfriend."

VI

Linda and I decided to put off any talk of moving for a while. So much had happened, we needed a break. We called a temporary cease-fire.

Out to dinner a month later, I overheard the conversation at a nearby table. The people seated behind us were psychiatric residents from USC, another of LA County's public mental health facilities. They were telling a gruesome story about a woman they'd admitted with no fingers, toes, ears or eyelids, who'd cut out her own tongue.

Linda caught my look of anguish. "Are you okay?"

I was a few seconds before I could speak. "She's someone I knew," I said, haltingly.

VII

I ran into Carlos Villegas at the video store. "How's the medication working?" I asked.

"Just fine, Dr. Seager," Carlos replied confidently.

VIII

A few months later, I got word that Lula Butts was back in the psych ER. When I arrived, she'd been heavily sedated and placed in restraints. Four security guards, ties askew and hair tousled, were just catching their breath. I checked Lula's room. Despite the medication she was still awake.

"Dr. Seager!" she said with a slur. "Come on over here, baby."

"Get some sleep." I turned off the light, went to the nursing station and started writing orders for her admission back to the ward.

IX

In all the commotion of the riots, Linda and the boys leaving and Jamal's hearing, I had forgotten to mail Tom Stanton's tin box and sympathy card to his parents. One afternoon, a couple in their sixties appeared at my office. They looked weary.

"We're Tom Stanton's parents," Mr. Stanton said. "You mentioned something about some of Tom's things?"

So much was suddenly going through my mind I could barely reply. "Come in," I said finally.

Opening a desk drawer, I pulled out the box and gave it to Mr. Stanton. It seemed like so little. "I have a card," I added. "The staff all signed it."

Mr. Stanton opened the envelope, then gave it to his wife.

"We're taking Tom back to Iowa," Mrs. Stanton said. "It's where he belongs."

It was too painful to speak for very long. We all shook hands and said goodbye. "Thank you," Mrs. Stanton said, taking my hand in both of hers.

Supported by the doorframe, I watched the Stantons slowly walk away.

X

I repaid Big John for the bus fare and phone money he'd given me. I mailed a check to the Safe Haven Rescue Mission for five hundred and one dollars and twenty-five cents.

XI

In September, Rev. Ike was murdered behind a nearby 7-11. I saw a small piece about it in the newspaper. There was no mention of a burial service.

XII

Recently, I came across another article in the local paper. "Identity of Homeless Man Remains a Mystery to Authorities" the headline read. The man, missing both legs and one arm, had been found three stories underground, clogging a main sewer pump. City officials became curious when the streets began to mysteriously flood. Inside his shirt pocket were two unfilled prescriptions from our psychiatric clinic.

Afterword

Solutions

What is to be done about the American system of care for the chronically mentally ill? Over the past years, I've read a great deal, discussed the issue with people in academics, the legal field and politics and have come to some conclusions about a solution. These aren't just my ideas but a collection of thoughts from many different sources. This final section includes a number of suggested actions for those bothered by the homeless mentally ill problem and interested in changing the way we treat people with disabling brain disease.

Number One: A Paradigm Shift

A paradigm is a basic model, an overall framework we use to explain and deal with a phenomenon. Our current, legally-weighted paradigm for the treatment of mental illness doesn't seem to be working. Perhaps a change is in order.

A change in thinking requires a new nomenclature. Schizophrenia, bipolar disorder, depression and all the other forms of mental illness—Tourette's disease, anxiety/panic, anorexia/bulimia and others—are, in fact, brain diseases, pathologic alterations in the organ's structure and function. AMI prefers the term brain disorder to mental illness. This designation seems more appropriate. It is akin to altering "mentally retarded" to "developmentally disabled" or "handicapped" to "physically challenged." It provides a keener, more accurate description of the process and affords an enhanced, compassionate assessment for those affected by the terminology.

There's no argument the "classic" brain maladies, e.g., Parkinson's disease, epilepsy, multiple sclerosis, Alzheimer's disease, Huntington's chorea and stroke, are biologically based. They produce obvious symptoms anyone can see—convulsions, paralysis, tremors and the like. It should be understood that the "mental" disorders are no different. They're also dysfunctions of the brain. Their symptoms, depression, anxiety, delusions and hallucinations, to name a few, are simply less obvious. You can't see them; the patient feels them. Nevertheless, they are all brain disorders.

Many people are susceptible to brain disorders. Twenty percent of women and twelve percent of men in the United States will suffer an episode of major depression at some point in their lives. One percent of the population is schizophrenic, and an equal number have bipolar disease. Three percent of the populace will come down with obsessive/compulsive disorder. Nearly six percent of us will suffer panic attacks, and eight percent must endure chronic, disabling anxiety. All in all, these are some serious numbers.

Brain disorders aren't mystical. Bad parenting or poor living conditions do not produce them. Moral or personal weakness plays no part in their genesis. You cannot talk or think your way into or out of them. Demons aren't to blame, nor is a "sick soul." These diseases aren't a punishment from God and don't result from sin. They are an "experience" but a bad one. We're not talking about a "life-style choice" or merely aberrant, irritating behavior. While useful on a metaphorical level—not unlike Greek myths—as an explanation for abnormal conduct, there's no such thing as a superego, ego or Id. Mental illness is a disease of the brain.

The most common misconception about brain disorders is that they are somehow caused by "stress." Everyone understands stress. For most of us, it is trouble at work, family conflicts, death of a loved one, financial pressure, etc. These problems don't cause brain disease. They can, however, make existing brain pathology worse or bring out an eruption of symptoms in someone already genetically predisposed. But this is the same for all diseases. Stress makes asthma, diabetes and high blood pressure worse as well, but no one claims it causes them.

Another misconception is that brain disorders aren't treatable. This simply isn't true. For many people, given the correct medication at an adequate dose for a long enough period of time, the symptoms of brain disease go away and life returns to normal.

Brain diseases act like all other diseases. They obey the "Rule of Thirds" that states that for any pathological process, given appropriate therapy, one-third of patients will improve completely and their problems never return; one-third will improve completely but suffer a relapse at some time in the future; and one-third will be chronically bothered by symptoms on a persistent basis. Heart disease works this way as do liver disease, cancer, brain disease and most major diseases. The bottom line is that sixty-six percent of people with brain disorders get better with treatment.

These concepts have been the subject of debate from time immemorial. The debate is over. Mental illness is brain disease, and it's treatable.

Number Two: Medical Insurance

A significant barrier for treating some brain disorders is a lack of medical insurance. Certain brain diseases, the mental illnesses, however, are not considered to be on par with other brain maladies. Most health care policies exclude them or offer minimal, substandard benefits. In the current managed care environment, many disorders are often "carved out." People with Alzheimer's disease are covered; people with schizophrenia are not. People with epilepsy are covered; people with bipolar disorder are not. You can visit the doctor as many times as necessary for heart trouble and diabetes, but severe limits are set for depression and anxiety. Without insurance, you can't get in the door of most hospitals, and many doctors won't give you an appointment.

It is often said that brain diseases are too expensive to treat, that they're chronic and disabling. Brain disorders are chronic and disabling mainly because they haven't been treated in the first place. Diabetes also leads to expensive disability if not cared for adequately, as do heart disease and hypertension. True, some schizophrenics never improve, but most do. No one with Alzheimer's *ever* gets better. Yet, patients with Alzheimer's are afforded care and dignity. The sickest schizophrenics die on the street.

What can we do? Every state has an insurance commissioner: think about writing or faxing him or her—ask for an answer. Medicare policy comes from Washington, Medicaid regulations from your state legislature. If you believe this situation is wrong, contact your federal or state representatives. Make your views known. Their telephone numbers are in the local directory.

Number Three: The Law

For many reasons, people who suffer from a specific class of brain disorders are seen as different in the eyes of the law. Many times they are judicially barred from receiving treatment and suffer atrocious depravation in the name of legal principle. Many people concerned with the brain disordered and their care seem to think that nothing can be done about the situation, that the "the law is the law." This position is erroneous. Laws are fluid. They can be altered as we see fit.

We have had unworkable laws before and corrected them. Prior to the 1860s, slavery was legal in many states. The Supreme Court authored the *Dred Scott* decision, affirming that institution. As well, in *Plessy v. Ferguson*, the same court coined the term "separate but equal," giving official sanction to segregation. These legal tenets were later thrown out. Ballot propositions have altered property tax laws and affirmative action programs. Capital punishment comes and goes.

In order to change the law, it is helpful to understand how laws are created. There are two ways. The first is called "Statutory Law." Legislative bodies generated these laws—the national Congress and Senate, as well as similar bodies at the state level. Bills are introduced that, when passed and signed by the President or Governor, become binding.

The second method is called "Case Law." These laws come from the courts. At the state and federal level, there are three tiers of jurisdiction. The first is the trial court. In California, this is known as the "Superior Court." Other states use different designations. Names aside, most of us are familiar with these proceedings. At the trial level, there is a judge and jury, testimony is given and arguments made. One side wins, the other loses.

If the defeated side appeals the decision, the case goes to the "Appellate Court." At this second rung, no new testimony or evidence is introduced. A three-judge panel reads the trial judge's decision and rules upon whether the trial was supervised properly. Incidentally, it is at this point that many defendants are released "on a technicality," i.e., there was an error in the way the trial was conducted.

For most cases that reach this second step, a written decision is issued by the Appellate Court stressing one or two key points of law around which the case revolved or explaining new interpretations of existing legal doctrines. This decision, or ruling, is also considered law. It sets a "precedent" that is binding statewide. The majority of mental health laws were produced in this way: no one voted for them, an appellate court ordered them.

What, then, can be done about mental health laws? They can be undone in exactly the same way they were generated. This means repealing existing statutes (the LPS Act in California, for example) and replacing them with new laws at the legislative level. This means contacting your legislators—senators, congresspersons, state representatives—and voicing your concerns. If enough people speak, they will listen.

Case law, as well, can be undone in the same manner it was produced. Anyone can file a lawsuit in defense of a brain-disordered person's right to adequate treatment. Remember, Roe had to sue Wade, and Brown had to bring action against the Little Rock Board of Education.

If we are going to change the laws and produce a new system of care for the chronically brain diseased, what should it look like? Specifically, what current laws need to be changed? What provisions should the new laws contain?

First, consider a change in the nature of involuntary commitment. New commitment standards should be written based upon medical, not primarily legal, considerations. These medical opinions would be generated in a cooperative, as opposed to adversarial, manner. Medical professionals, the patient, the patient's family and a citizens panel could meet and decide what will best promote a person's return to well-being. The decision should be made early in a patient's commitment, thus alleviating long delays and repetitive reviews. A decision to treat should never hinge upon whether a sick person has twenty dollars and knows the address of a public shelter.

As well, an equally important but probably necessary matter would be removing the court's involvement in the day-to-day running of a psychiatric ward. Treatment and detainment decisions could be made on more compassionate grounds by a citizens panel. The courts would, of course, continue to monitor patients' living conditions to ensure the abuses of the past never recur.

In the psychiatric literature this is called "A Need for Treatment" model. It is an idea worth thinking about.

Second, a new version of commitment itself could be developed. Treatment of brain disease doesn't always have to be given in a hospital. Outpatient care works for many people, but most of the severely brain diseased refuse it, and the law currently supports them in this decision, sanctioning often dangerous and demented people to skip doctor's appointments, refuse medication and live in the streets.

This problem could be at least partially alleviated by a concept called "Outpatient Commitment," in which follow-up doctor visits and medication compliance are legally mandated. If dangerous, disastrously sick people want to live in the community, they must take their medication. A mental health outreach team could investigate missed appointments. Non-compliance with medication intake leading to continued psychosis would mandate rehospitalization.

Some states already have outpatient commitment laws on the books. In Dane County, Wisconsin, such laws resulted in a seventy-five percent drop in rehospitalization rates. Overall, this could be a cheaper and more humane solution for many people, maximizing a sick person's chance to get well while being fiscally responsible.

The idea of mandated treatment isn't so unusual. Alzheimer's patients don't wander the streets. Many communicable diseases can be quarantined. There are current laws requiring treatment of tuberculosis including involuntary rehospitalization for medication refusal. In old English common law, this precept was known as "assisted treatment."

Third, we should consider a change in the way due process applies to the treatment of brain disease. The unfortunate results of *Lessard v. Schmidt* and its "criminalization" of commitment proceedings might be reconsidered. This has already begun in the California prison system. In *Washington v. Harper*, an appellate court ruled that due process could be served by an internal administrative review of treatment decisions for brain-diseased inmates, not a judicial one. In effect, persons other than the court can decide such matters. This gives legal precedent to the notion of citizens panels.

Other legal doctrines might need readjustments as well. There's a pervasive tenet in current mental health law called "Least Restrictive Alternative." This states that a person should be treated in the environment that allows him the most personal freedom. In theory, this doesn't sound bad. In practice, however, it often means living on the street as this, of course, is the least restrictive alternative of all. A new doctrine, "The Most Therapeutic Alternative," might take its place. The streets and public shelters should be dropped from the list of "alternatives" entirely. Personal freedom is important. When dementia, rape, murder and starvation are the result, however, safety, protection and treatment probably should supersede.

As importantly, we might think about changing the arbitrarily determined length of involuntary commitments, e.g., fourteen days in California. A person's stay in an institution, in-patient or out, should be based on therapeutic indications, not a randomly set limit. Remember, in the 1890s, if patients were initially held for three to nine months, more than half of them never needed hospitalization again. The course of their disease was changed for good. This alone could dramatically improve the lives of millions of people and perhaps prevent many of them from suffering the debilitating effects of chronic disease and the concomitant terrors of neglect and abuse.

The issue of treatment refusal during involuntary detainment deserves revision as well. The idea of court-ordered warehousing makes little sense. A new system might include something like the aforementioned Utah statute. After a psychiatric evaluation, if involuntary treatment is required, this would be *prima facie* evidence of diminished competence. An incompetent person shouldn't be making treatment decisions.

Finally, the current commitment standards in many states are woefully low. "Surviving" on the street for those who are sick is a questionable ideal, at best. Being able to provide for food, clothing and shelter, when food comes from a garbage pile, clothing is a hospital gown and adequate shelter is defined as lying underneath a car, isn't enough. Perhaps a more humane standard can be adopted, one that includes living in a clean facility, eating healthy food and wearing decent clothing.

A modern, medically based, comprehensive plan for treatment of the brain diseased appears to be more in line with what people want and need. Personal rights deserve protection, and abuses need to be prevented, but the over-arching concern, perhaps, should be compassionate and personalized care arrived at by a consensus.

Even Frank Lanterman, co-author of the original Lanterman-Petris-Short Act, in one of his last interviews expressed his horror about the current mental health system. His secretary Elaine Dewees was quoted in the December 5, 1987 edition of the *LA Times*, saying: "One of Frank's and my last conversations is burned deeply in my memory. Frank Lanterman, the irascible curmudgeon with a heart of gold, had tears in his eyes when he said, 'I wanted the LPS Act to help the mentally ill. I never meant for it to prevent those who need care from receiving it. The law has to be changed.'" As Rael Isaac and D.J. Jaffe said in a 1996 *National Review* article: "Mental illness is not a lifestyle; it is a disease that can lead to homelessness, violence and death. But it can often be treated especially when the law isn't in the way."

Number Four: State Hospitals

The deinstitutionalization of the brain disordered, while well intentioned, has proven to be less than successful. It has devolved into what's known as "De-population." The hospitals were simply closed, and their patients, most in dire need of continuing care, released to fend for themselves. Most ended up on the street. On some level, the state hospitals—a single focus of comprehensive treatment and shelter for the most severely brain diseased—should be reinstituted. In the 1950s and 1960s, had these facilities been reformed rather than dismantled, some of the problems we face today might have been avoided.

Given an adequate outpatient system with guaranteed, quality care, most brain diseased individuals can live in the community. But some cannot. For those whose brains have been so severely damaged by disease, complete management appears to be the only option. This is what state hospitals provide.

Smaller local facilities might also be substituted. The theory remains the same: long-term patient care and stabilization.

Number Five: Money

Major change costs money and revamping the care delivery system for the chronically brain disordered will initially seem expensive. Facilities will need to be constructed or reconfigured and staff hired. Medications have to be purchased. But the task will not be as onerous as you might think. Simply removing the brain disordered from the prison systems (thirty thousand in California alone) would probably offset any monetary outlay. Carla Jacobs, board member of the California Alliance for the Mentally Ill, has figures that say that untreated brain disorders cost the state of California 1.2 to 1.8 billion dollars per year in criminal justice costs alone. There are no adequate estimates available, but decreasing court costs as well as police time would probably generate significant savings.

With adequate initial treatment, a significant amount of long-term psychiatric disability might be prevented, which would be cheaper in the long run.

But this is not, at its core, a money question. It is a "do-the-right-thing" issue. Americans have traditionally taken care of the poor and disadvantaged. It is in our nature. We authored Medicare, the Head Start program and Aid-to-Dependent-Children.

We can tackle this problem too.

Number Six: Public Safety

A fact long suspected but only recently documented, is that people with untreated brain disease are significantly more violent than the general population. This is an issue AMI has always tried to downplay, thinking it "stigmatizes" the patient. But now, stigma or no, the verdict is in.

Of patients recently discharged from psychiatric hospitals, twenty-seven percent commit a violent act within four months. Unmedicated schizophrenics use weapons in fights twenty-one times more frequently than those without brain disorders. In metropolitan areas, two-thirds of people who pushed or tried to push another person onto a subway track had inadequately treated brain disease.

There are three proven predictors of violence: a past history of brutality, drug use and unmedicated brain disorder. As John Monahan of the University of Virginia Law School writes: "The data that have recently become available, fairly read, suggest the one conclusion I did not want to reach... Mental disorder may be a robust and significant risk factor for the occurrence of violence."

The conclusion strengthens an argument for enforced treatment. In this particular instance, public safety appears to be a "greater good" than personal rights.

Number Seven: A Moral Issue

Allowing our brothers and sisters, parents and children with brain sickness—demented and delusional, fetid and starving—to live in our streets and sewers feels wrong. For them to languish in prisons is equally disquieting. Most people are familiar with the mentally ill person on the street; those in jail are not so visible, but their living conditions are equally deplorable. I again quote Carla Jacobs, board member of California Alliance for the Mentally Ill: "Our family members frequently are locked in the SHU, a secluded housing unit, designed for punishment. Small six-by-seven holes, they are locked up for twenty-two and one-half hours per day; they never see direct sunlight or, for the most part, other prisoners, let alone doctors, patient advocates or nurses. Or, if that isn't degrading enough, they are moved to the VCU, Violence Control Unit, where discipline includes denying them basic necessities. VCU prisoners are denied bedding, cups to drink from, eating utensils. They are left handcuffed and hog-tied, forcing them to lap their food from their plates like dogs. Rarely are they given medication or treatment. These are conditions worse than the worst hellholes of old. How has this happened?"

The situation is somewhat similar to that of segregation prior to the 1960s. As long as people argued the reasons for or against this venal institution, there was no progress. It wasn't until Dr. Martin Luther King elevated the issue to a moral plane that we saw results. No matter the reason, he argued, segregation and second-class treatment based upon race is wrong. It is the same with our treatment of the homeless and incarcerated mentally ill. It is just wrong.

And, if asked, the current system is not really what most people want. People do care. They simply don't know what to do. Many believe there are no other options. Of course, this isn't so. There is another way to do things.

Number Eight: What to Do First

This one is easier. Become aware. Become involved. Many of you have brain-diseased relatives or friends, some lost to the hard streets. Make people familiar with the problem. Talk to your friends. Provide them with literature. Use the media at every opportunity to spread the word. Make treatment for the chronically brain diseased part of the national agenda again.

Contact your local, state and federal representatives. Write letters suggesting they author or support new brain disease treatment legislation. Question legislative candidates about their views on brain disease. Ask how they plan to change things.

Join the Alliance for the Mentally Ill in your community. The local number is in every phone book. The national office in Arlington,
Virginia can be reached at (703) 524-7600. Realize how many families are suffering because of the way our current mental health system
is constructed. Become aware of the personal toll we are exacting on
our weakest citizens. Do something about it.

A Final Note: Other Countries

Deinstitutionalization of the chronically mentally ill is currently
unique to the United States. Many other countries, however, are con-
sidering a similar move. To these governments a word of caution is in
order: If community care for the seriously brain diseased is the path
upon which you want to travel, do so carefully. It hasn't worked well
here.

Order Form

❏ Yes! Please send me *Street Crazy, The Tragedy of the Homeless Mentally Ill*

Name _____ _____

Address _____ _____

City _____State _____Zip _____

Phone _____Fax_____ _____

Email_____

Book Title	Qty.	Cost Ea.	Total
Street Crazy, The Tragedy	_____	$12.95	_____
of the Homeless Mentally Ill		Subtotal	_____
(CA residents add 8.25%)		Tax	_____
($3.25 for 1st book, $2 for ea. additional)		Shipping	_____
		TOTAL	$ _____

Mail order and make check payable to:
    WESTCOM PRESS
    2110 Artesia Boulevard, Suite 183
    Redondo Beach, CA 90278

VISA   MasterCard

Visa and MasterCard accepted

Card # _____ Exp date ___ /___

Phone: (310) 374-0988 OR Fax: (310) 371-8244

Web Address: http://www.StreetCrazy.com

Call for quantity discounts